TH

TAO

OF

BEAUTY

BROADWAY BOOKS   *New York*

THE TAO OF BEAUTY

Chinese Herbal Secrets to Feeling Good and Looking Great

HELEN LEE

This book is dedicated to my mother, who guided me with her deep wisdom and always encouraged me. She is the most loving and caring person I know, giving to all in need without expecting any recognition or reward.

My goal is to be as great a person as she and as good a mother to my daughter, Samantha, who gives me my greatest joy.

BROADWAY

THE TAO OF BEAUTY. Copyright © 1999 by Helen Lee. All rights reserved. Printed in the United States of America. No part of this book may be reproduced or transmitted in any form or by any means, electronic or mechanical, including photocopying, recording, or by any information storage and retrieval system, without written permission from the publisher. For information, address Broadway Books, a division of Random House, Inc., 1540 Broadway, New York, NY 10036.

Broadway Books titles may be purchased for business or promotional use or for special sales. For information, please write to: Special Markets Department, Random House, Inc., 1540 Broadway, New York, NY 10036.

BROADWAY BOOKS and its logo, a letter B bisected on the diagonal, are trademarks of Broadway Books, a division of Random House, Inc.

Library of Congress Cataloging-in-Publication Data
Lee, Helen, 1958–
The Tao of beauty : Chinese herbal secrets to feeling good and looking great / Helen Lee. — 1st ed.
p.   cm.
Includes bibliographical references and index.
ISBN 0-7679-0256-4 (pbk.)
1. Women—Health and hygiene.   2. Beauty, Personal.   3. Medicine, Chinese.   4. Herbal cosmetics.
5. Herbs—Therapeutic use.
I. Title.
RA778.L4625   1999
613'.04243—dc21   98-31738
                                                                              CIP
ISBN-13: 978-0-7679-0256-4

The epigraph on page ix is excerpted from *The Illustrated Tao Te Ching*. Copyright © Man-Ho Kwok, Martin Palmer, Jay Ramsey, 1993. Used by permission of Element Books, Inc., Boston, Massachusetts.

FIRST EDITION

Designed by Jennifer Daddio and Ralph Fowler
Illustrations by The Strausberg Group (botanicals) and Cathy Pavia (Chi Gung)

00   01   02   03   10   9   8   7   6   5   4   3   2

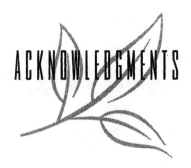

ACKNOWLEDGMENTS

I wish to thank my mother, all my sisters—Betty, Doris, Fanny, Janice, Lisa, and Robin—and my brother, Tim, as well as my late father, for sharing their knowledge, providing references, and giving support and encouragement, especially when I needed it most. Thanks to Dr. Jie He Li, Dr. Yue Chan, and Dr. James Ji, who were wonderful advisors and teachers. I also wish to thank my husband, Lance, for his help, advice, and support. This book would not have been possible without them.

Thanks to all the staff of the Helen Lee Spa, particularly my manager, Tina, and assistant, Arlene, for their help. I also wish to thank the spa clients who contributed to this book. My friends Cydna Moore, George Sing, George Fan, Peter Regna, Scott Shellstrom, Steve Prezant, Steve Forrest, and Joe Zaino, were always there when I needed them.

A special thanks to my agent, Katharine Sands, who helped in so many ways to make this book possible, and to Sallie Batson for her help in writing the text; Kimberly Blackwood for helping with the recipes and for her writing assistance.

Thanks to Tracy Behar, my editor, for believing in me and for having the understanding and vision for this book . . . and for all her time and patience. This book would never have been possible without the guidance, editorial support, understanding, and patience of Tracy and her assistant, Angela Casey, of Broadway Books.

CONTENTS

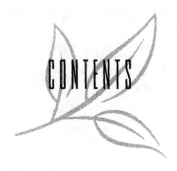

The Tao

                    is the breath that never dies.

It is a Mother to All Creation.

It is the root and ground of every soul

—the fountain of Heaven and Earth, laid open.

                    Endless source, endless river

                    River of no shape, river of no water

                    Drifting invisibly from place to place

. . . it never ends

                    and it never fails.

                                        LAO TZU

NOTE FROM THE AUTHOR

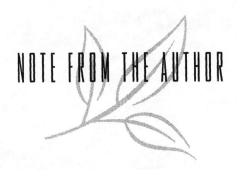

Many Western people have difficulty in understanding the Chinese philosophy of health and beauty. Writing this book has given me a genuine appreciation for having this ancient philosophy as an integral part of my upbringing. As an adult I was inspired to study Chinese herbal medicine formally so that I could broaden and deepen my knowledge and understanding. I moved to the United States in my early teens, so I was exposed to the ways of the West at a relatively early age. By experiencing both Eastern and Western cultures, I have gained an appreciation and respect for what each has to offer. These two philosophies are very different, and it is my hope that I increase your understanding.

The Tao of Beauty is a primer of the most basic and general information on Chinese concepts of health and beauty, made relevant and accessible for the modern woman.

Please read this book with an open mind. Our bodies are miraculous. Depending on how we nourish and care for them, they can heal themselves as well as produce toxins and spread disease. The Chinese concept starts with prevention, then emphasizes proper nourishment to attain balance. Harmony and balance are in every aspect of our lives. It is my hope that this book will help you on the path to a healthier, more beautiful, and happier life. Enjoy.

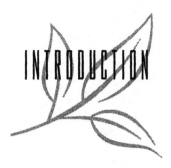

INTRODUCTION

All of us know of women who are *beautiful* but would hardly be considered *pretty*. Their eyes may be "too small" or "too far apart" or their nose or lips "too large" or their figures far from ideal. Yet they have something extra, magnetic—something from within—that renders them beautiful. How is it that they possess this quality that can only be called a glow?

According to Chinese tradition, the path, or *Tao* (pronounced "dow"), of beauty is simply one lane on the road to radiant health. There is nothing particularly unusual about this. Health is beauty; beauty is health. No amount of makeup can camouflage a body that isn't healthy or, as we Chinese view it, is out of balance.

This often comes as a surprise to new clients who come into my day spa expecting a facial, instruction in skin care, and a makeup application. The nutritional aspects of the beauty program that I offer are deeply rooted in the practices of traditional Chinese medicine. To the Chinese, the term "medicine" relates to a way to healthy life rather than to treatment for illness. These concepts are very different from Western beauty culture.

While cosmetics and skin care can enhance a woman's outer appearance, real beauty must be solidly based in balance and health. Strong, glossy hair; clear, bright eyes; firm, glowing skin; and strong, pink fingernails—these are the foundations that makeup merely plays up. Nothing can be enhanced that isn't intrinsically there. This is why the road to beauty, as outlined in this book, is inextricably linked to optimal health.

Our bodies are in a constant state of renewal. Old cells die as new ones are born. By properly nourishing these cells, we can insure that we grow healthier, stronger, and consequently more beautiful day by day.

In my experience as a Ford fashion model as well as in my spa, I have found that many of the most beautiful women are those who have created their own beauty-wellness programs based on this philosophy of balance. No matter how busy we are, to regenerate our bodies and refresh our spirits is a gift we give not only to ourselves but to those we love as well. As the old Chinese proverb states, "An empty well gives no water." When we take time—even if it's just a few moments a day—to revitalize ourselves, we have so much more to share with those around us.

The Tao of Beauty offers more than a frantic shape-up plan of diet, exercise, and makeup tricks. It provides a foundation of practices and recipes for balance and wellness that will fortify your body for health and beauty. As so many of us have learned, quick fixes are usually transient, lasting only until the pressure of our everyday lives takes precedence over our best intentions. I will give you in clear, precise language a life path, or Tao, so you can release the power of your beauty and serenity.

My ancestors were Chinese healers and herbalists, and I draw upon this heritage to share the ancient philosophy of Tao. First, I will show you how to determine your basic type according to Chinese principles—yin, yang, or yin/yang (balanced)—and you will then be able to fashion your own beauty-wellness program. I'll show you how to draw from a full range of simple, easy-to-prepare recipes for delicious foods to eat, teas to drink, and potions to apply to your body to obtain the beautiful results you desire.

Unlike conventional Western beauty, diet, and exercise books that mandate a step-by-step routine to be followed to the letter for specific results, *The Tao of Beauty* offers a program that you can adapt to meet your body's needs. You will learn to be in touch with how you feel and what your body needs to correct or maintain the delicate balance of its life energy, or *chi*.

As a busy working mother, I can fully appreciate that time is always in short supply. With this in mind, I have made sure that the program you design for yourself and the recipes you use are simple to follow. Most of the ingredients for this newfound Tao are either already in your kitchen or in your corner supermarket. For example, you'll find two powerful food-grade herbs with strong healing properties, *xiohuixiang* and *dingxiang*, masquerading under the names fennel and cloves, respectively. Some Asian herbs, like ginseng and royal jelly, are already known in the West. These, and many items that are less familiar, such as dang quai and dried Chinese red dates, can be inexpensively purchased in many well-stocked health food stores. I've also listed mail-order sources in the back of this book for your convenience. Furthermore, I've made sure that the recipes require minimal cooking skill and little more equipment than a blender, a few enamel and glass pots and pans, and a few glass bowls.

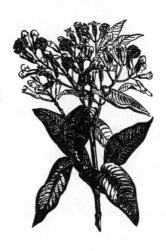

Clove tree *(Syzygium aromticum)*

I invite you now to join me on this radiant path. Put aside everything you already know about your body; suspend your beliefs about how you should look and what is beautiful. I will introduce you to a new way of thinking that is, in truth, centuries old.

BEAUTY
BEGINS
WITH
HEALTH

1.

BALANCE IS BEAUTY, BEAUTY IS HEALTH

UNDERSTANDING THE TAO OF BEAUTY

For centuries, the study of Chinese herbal medicine has included beauty as one of the results of good health. The concepts of health and beauty are inseparable, focusing on the total well-being of the body's internal and external functions. To have optimum health and beauty, a great physique and youthful appearance has to start with the body's inner health, which includes maintaining the balance of *yin* and *yang, chi,* and blood action.

To get the most out of *The Tao of Beauty,* it is important to understand the underlying principles that inform Chinese thought. Whether we are talking about health or the weather, several important concepts apply. At the top of this list is the principle of the Organic Whole, followed by the theory of Yin and Yang. In addition, there are *chi* or life force, the Five Elements, nature's Six Climatic Effects, and the Five Emotions.

Using these special points as an outline for your new venture, I promise that you'll soon be in touch with your body—and your beauty—like never before.

A BRIEF HISTORY OF CHINESE MEDICINE

I come from a family of herbalists, and I've heard stories since childhood about the amazing work done by such great pioneers as Emperor Shen Nong, who introduced agriculture to the Chinese people around 3000 B.C.E. According to legend, Shen Nong was intrigued by the vast numbers and varieties of plants around him and began to experiment with herbs. As the first in a long line of Chinese herbal "explorers," he and his disciples tested thousands of these plants—tasting them, cooking them, and making teas from them. In the process of this delicate, dedicated study, they discovered through shrewd and careful observation, that many of these plants not only tasted good but also enabled people to stay vigorous and strong. The vast variety and effects of these herbs was a challenge to Shen Nong and the long line of others who followed him in this quest. Some herbs induced sleep, others wakefulness; still others eased pain or helped people recover quickly from even the most serious illnesses. They also found that some made the skin soft and beautiful and others enhanced youth and vitality.

These formulations were passed down through the generations and refined until, centuries later, during the reign of Huang Di of the Han dynasty (206 B.C.E.–220 C.E.), this knowledge was collected and incorporated into a book entitled *The Yellow Emperor's Classic Book of Medicine*. This is generally recognized as one of the first known formal Chinese medical texts.

My mother, who comes from a long line of Chinese herbalists, is an ardent believer in traditional Chinese medicine. She served my family foods that were in season to maintain balance within us; this kept us healthy and strong. Instead of going to the pharmacy for pills if we were ill, she cooked special dishes that were known to treat whatever was out of balance within us. She brewed special herbal tonics that would strengthen our immune systems or speed up our recovery by helping our bodies renew their internal balance. She also prepared toners, bath salts, and other topical treatments that affected our total well-being and promoted beautiful, glowing skin and strong, shining hair.

Few things are more effective than Chinese herbal formulas to maintain balance in the human body. I will show you that a complete beauty regimen can be based on a well-balanced nutritional program designed to provide a foundation of health. This high level of health provides the groundwork for natural beauty and prevention of disease. Western medicine is great for acute intervention—X rays for broken bones, surgery, diagnostics, and so on—but it doesn't address total wellness from this traditional Chinese perspective.

By the time you've finished this book, you'll be figuring out what foods you need to bring equilibrium or balance to your system. You will incorporate common foods into your diet with natural awareness that they are nourishing your body at a cellular level, encouraging your hair to grow without graying, cleansing your body so that it becomes free of age-causing toxins, even making your fingernails grow long and strong.

The starting place for any study of this ancient practice is a concept we call the Organic Whole.

THE ORGANIC WHOLE

All life is part of nature—an organic whole that includes the earth and the cosmos. Notice that I said "part of nature," as in part of a whole.

When the weather turns cold, we know that we need to wear more clothing to stay warm. During winter, we eat heavier, more filling foods—root vegetables, hot soups, and the like—that warm our bodies from the inside out, as opposed to summer, when we eat lighter, cooling foods. During hot weather we need more cooling liquids and foods with a high moisture content to replenish the fluids lost through perspiration. Nature supplies us with juice-filled fruits and melons to make it easier for us to meet this need.

Nature is always in and around us. The seas and trees supply us with the oxygen we inhale to sustain life. In turn, we exhale carbon dioxide, which trees and other plants need for photosynthesis. When we are in harmony with the natural rhythms of nature, we experience a sense of health and well-being. When we oppose these forces, we are edgy, uncomfortable, and in extreme cases, ill. Premature aging can also result from imbalances in our bodies.

When I was flying back and forth between New York and Paris, New York and Rome, Rome and Hong Kong, Hong Kong and New York on modeling assignments, my body's "timeclock" was constantly upset as I raced from time zone to time zone. My sleep was so disrupted that I often woke up from a nap exhausted. I was always tired, no matter how much I slept, dehydrated from spending so much time in the pressurized environment of airplanes. And hungry. Really hungry. The balanced, healthy way of eating that my mother had taught me was ignored. It was too old-fashioned for me at that time. After all, I was a modern girl.

I loved my life as an international fashion model, but before long, my looks began to suffer. My hair lost its luster, and my skin was dry and flaking in some areas and tender with acne in others. I had absolutely no energy. I was out of harmony, out of balance. And my body showed it. I went to a series of Western doctors who treated me with antibiotics and injections. My skin would clear up, but recovery was always short-lived, so back to the doctor I'd go. Obviously, with my face breaking out, I was unable to work, so I took time to visit my parents, who were then living in Arizona. My mother immediately began to feed me the foods and tonics my body needed to heal itself and prepared soothing masks and toners to ease the blemishes and pain that were plaguing my skin. Within a week or two, the redness and flaking began to subside and my energy returned. Soon, as balance was restored to my body and my *chi* was flowing freely, I was my lively, clear-skinned self again.

When we speak of the Organic Whole and the principles of yin and yang, we must remember that these laws are not absolute. In fact, they are quite changeable, just like the weather and the world around us. We've all had days that started out at an easygoing, balanced pace, only to have everything erupt with hot yang anger when the flight to the Caribbean was missed, or everything screeched to a halt when a very yin snowstorm blanketed the city. By being aware of the potential for changes that can disrupt the balance of our bodies and our lives, we are able to maintain a higher level of wellness and beauty.

YIN AND YANG

In the process of all this research, ancient Chinese scholars formulated what is known as the "Theory of Opposing Principles." Simply put, all forces of nature have two equal yet opposing—and very necessary—sides: deficiency and excess, cold and hot, recessive and dominant, negative and positive, dark and light. Yin and yang represent these two fundamental universal forces. When these equal, interdependent components are in balance, optimal movement of the life force—*chi,* or *qi,* pronounced "chee"—is possible. Yin energy moves inward and downward, affecting internal organs and body fluids. Yang energy moves upward and outward, toward the surface of the body.

When these forces are in harmony, there is balance. When there is balance, there is optimum health. Where there is optimum health, there is amazing beauty. This occurs when yin and yang are in harmony.

Chinese doctors have traditionally concentrated on keeping these forces balanced in their patients. When yin and yang are in sync, harmony (and thus good health and beauty) prevails. Unlike Western doctors who concentrate on the treatment of illness, Chinese physicians are trained to focus on the wellness of their patients. A good Chinese doctor has only well patients.

Harmony and balance are woven throughout nature so strongly that they make up the cultural fabric of Chinese civilization itself. Even the most humble housewife keeps these ideas in mind while preparing her family's daily meals.

You have probably been practicing the yin/yang concept already—it's a supremely natural way to live. For example, hot days (yang) require cooling foods (yin). This is why watermelon tastes so good in the summer—it balances the heat that you feel in the environment and within your own body. Cold days (yin) require warming foods (yang). Few things are better than a steaming bowl of spicy chicken soup or beef stew in the dead of winter.

The Chinese characters for yin and yang present vivid images of their meanings. The character for yin means "shadow" or without sun, "the shady side of the mountain," while the character for yang means "sun," as in "the sunny side of the mountain." Yin is cold or cool and calm, and yang is hot and active. The upper part of the human body is yang and the lower part, yin; the exterior is yang and the interior is yin; the back—which gets sunburned more often—is yang and the front, yin. Your arms, which are yang in nature, as they are extensions of the upper part of the body, also have their yin and yang sides. When you drop your arms to your sides, you will notice that the outside is exposed to the sun, while the inside, which lies against your torso, is not. The outside is yang; the inside, yin.

All life can be divided into equal yet opposing yin and yang forces. The attraction or repulsion of these opposing forces, like the alternating of electrical charges from positive to negative and back, or the action of two toy magnets, makes movement and change possible. This movement provides the underlying life energy, *chi,* in *all* life. Yin energy is passive and slow moving, while yang energy is active and fast moving. Yin and yang may cause the movement of *chi,* but it's up to us to maintain and control the flow of that force as it moves through our bodies.

Once you become aware of this, you'll find yourself automatically identifying which energy and which activities are yin in nature, and which are yang. Quietness is obviously yin, while loudness is yang; peace and stability are yin; war and activity are yang. Cold energy is yin; hot is yang.

All living beings, our bodies included, are in a constant state of change, made possible by the yin/yang interaction. Many factors contribute to change—what we eat, our level of activity or inactivity, job stress, even the weather. While we can be yin today or yang tomorrow, we generally follow a pattern, falling more often into one or the other category.

CHI—LIFE'S ENERGY

At the heart of the Tao of beauty is the life force we call *chi.* Although every form of traditional medicine shares the concept of a living energy that sustains all life, the term *chi* has no true English-language equivalent. The Japanese refer to this force as *ki,* while Hindus call it *prana.* The Greek term is *pneuma.*

In Chinese medicine *chi* is interpreted in two ways: internally and externally. Internally, it's one of the three substances that enable the organs to function; the other two are blood and bodily fluids. Externally, *chi* is taken in through metabolic nourishment, which is carried by food and water.

Chi moves in the body through a network of channels, or meridians, that govern how the body functions, much like an irrigation system that carries water to a field. These meridians form a network through which *chi* courses to empower every organ in the body. When energy is blocked or slowed as it travels through these channels, organs, tissues, and even cells are deprived of the power needed to function at top potential. Even one block in the flow of *chi* can cause the whole organism to malfunction.

ACUPUNCTURE, ACUPRESSURE, AND EXERCISE

Chinese scholars have studied the meridians for thousands of years, developing the healing art we now know as acupuncture, and its related therapy, acupressure, to disperse energy blockages and restore balance. The acupuncturist inserts fine needles in the appropriate meridians to free blocked energy so that *chi* can move freely, while the acupressure practitioner presses and manipulates points on the body to encourage the flow of *chi*.

Exercises that manipulate the flow of *chi* have been practiced in a variety of forms for thousands of years. The Chinese exercise called *Chi Kung*—*chi,* meaning "energy," as well as "breath" and "air," and *kung* meaning "work" or "skill"— began as a therapeutic dance to ward off rheumatism and other symptoms of illness. Through the ages, it evolved into a complete energy management program of meditative breathing, concentrated movements, and martial arts. I'll teach you the basic *Chi Kung* exercises I learned from my parents in Chapter 10, Exercises for Energy (page 187). These exercises direct the flow of *chi* through the meridians and energize the body.

There are twelve main meridians, each relating to specific organs in the body. Branching from there is a complex network of supplementary channels, of which the smallest, cutaneous, meridians run just under the skin. There are approximately 365 acupuncture points, or energy vortices, along the main channels, with many more along the smaller channels. These points are places where the flow of *chi* is frequently disrupted. Generally, they are found at indentations or bumps in the path, such as where two muscles intersect, where there is a notch in a bone, or at a joint.

While meridians are not visible to the human eye, they can often be felt. For example, there is a point in the mound of tissue between your thumb and forefinger that will get rid of headaches. With the thumb and forefinger of your right hand, locate the point where your thumb connects with the bones of the forefinger of your left hand, then move back just a little bit into the web of flesh. If you have a headache you will invariably hit a tender spot. That spot is the blocked meridian. Press gently and massage this spot for a minute. Release the pressure and switch hands, using the thumb and forefinger of your left hand to massage the meridian on your right hand. Within another minute or two, you should begin to feel relief from your headache. (NOTE: This exercise is not recommended for pregnant women.)

THE FOUR TYPES OF CHI

There are four types of *chi*—inborn or original, pectoral, nourishing, and defending.

1. **Inborn or original *chi*.**   This is the life force we inherit from our parents. It is the most fundamental form of *chi*, and it is stored in the kidneys.
2. **Pectoral *chi*.**   This is derived primarily from the air we breathe. This *chi* is stored in the lungs.
3. **Nourishing *chi*.**   This energy is essential to replenish and revitalize the tissues of the body. Derived from food and water, this life force circulates through the bloodstream.
4. **Defending *chi*.**   This external energy force protects the body from hostile conditions such as inclement weather or even germs, while maintaining body temperature by controlling the opening and closing of pores. Think of this as an external force field surrounding and protecting your body.

When flows freely through the channels or meridians, we experience not only health and vitality but also full expression of our inner selves.

HOW CHI WORKS

Chi has five primary functions. Although they are very different, they are closely related. They serve to keep the body operating efficiently and healthily.

1. **Growing action.**   According to the Chinese way of thinking, the initial *chi* function is growth. *Chi* is the primary source of energy responsible

🌿 BEAUTY BEGINS WITH HEALTH

for growth and development of the body. Lack of *chi* can result in delayed or slow physical and mental development, insufficient blood formation, weak digestion and bowel function, low energy, or disturbed metabolism. In terms of beauty, this results in weak, short nails, thin hair, and increased hair loss, as well as loss of skin color and tone.

2. **Warming action.** *Chi* is the main source of body heat, which maintains the health of the organs. Lack of *chi* can cause intolerance to cold, especially in the limbs. It can also cause purple lips and runny noses. When *chi* is flowing properly, your cheeks will be rosy and your lips pink.

3. **Defending action.** *Chi* protects the body from invasion of toxins by guarding the surface of the skin. Without sufficient defensive *chi,* you can develop itching, eczema, or other topical skin irritations.

4. **Governing action.** *Chi* maintains the movement of all fluids throughout the body, from blood, perspiration, and saliva to sperm, urination, and excretion. It keeps your blood flowing and controls glandular secretions. Governing action also prevents organs from descending. Poor governing *chi* can cause water retention and weight gain.

5. **Transforming action.** *Chi* performs actions that affect the body's metabolism, causing changes within the body. This energy relates to the vital energy of blood and fluids, as well as the digestion of food, transforming the essence of the food into the energy the body needs.

The Tao of beauty calls for us to maintain maximum flow of *chi.* As you will soon learn, there are many simple ways to do this, mostly by using herbs and foods that have been found to restore balance throughout the body, and by cultivating the breathing and exercise techniques associated with the practice of *Chi Kung,* detailed in Chapter 10.

THE FIVE ELEMENTS

One of the fundamentals of traditional Chinese philosophies, including medicine and, consequently, of the Tao of beauty, is the theory of the Five Elements—

wood, fire, earth, metal, and water. Identified by ancient scholars as essential to sustaining life, these substances provided a matrix for all life.

Applied to the seasonal cycles, wood is equated with spring; fire, summer; earth, late summer; metal, autumn; and water, winter. This concept comes directly from ancient Chinese healers who determined that *chi* moves throughout nature—including our bodies—in a rhythmic, orderly, continuous circuit. These great healers also identified the relationship between the Five Elements and the organs of our bodies.

Just as we are born under specific astrological signs that reflect our personalities, our organs have their own chart related to the Five Elements. We have five main organ groups that correspond to the Five Elements. Each organ group consists of one yin organ and one yang organ; yin organs are solid, while yang organs are hollow. The liver (yin) and gallbladder (yang) are associated with the wood element; the heart (yin) and the small intestine (yang) are associated with fire; the spleen and pancreas (yin) and stomach (yang) are associated with earth; the lungs (yin) and the large intestine (yang) are associated with metal; and the kidneys (yin) and bladder (yang) are associated with water. See page 29 for a chart that summarizes the way the Chinese view the human body.

The Five Elements represent the five stages that are characteristic to *all change*. By understanding this concept, we can understand how to restore the yin/yang balance within our bodies and maintain the health and beauty of the Organic Whole.

HOW ENERGY FLOWS THROUGH THE FIVE ELEMENTS AND THEIR CORRESPONDING ORGAN GROUPS

The circular diagram below illustrates how the nurturing energy of the Five Elements and their corresponding organ groups flows from one element to the other in a "creative" or energy-generating cycle, while the star-shaped diagram shows the controlling or limiting properties of these same elements and organ groups. Like the relationship between mother and child, the elements nurture each other. On the other hand, each element also has the disciplinary quality of a father-child relationship. I'll do my best to explain the energy flow between the Five Elements as simply as possible.

Starting with wood, follow me around the circle:

- Wood burns, or nurtures fire. Once burned, ashes become part of the earth.
- Therefore, fire generates earth.
- Earth—the source of ore—generates metal.
- Metal—or minerals—dissolve in and therefore empower water.
- Water keeps trees—wood—alive.

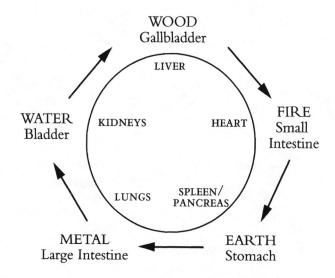

The Nurturing Energy Among the Five Elements and their corresponding organs
NOTE: *Yang organs are on the outside of the circle; yin organs on the inside.*

Now follow me through the star diagram, which demonstrates how the elements control or restrict one another.

- Metal controls or restricts wood, as an axe will cut a tree.
- Wood restricts earth, as the root of a tree will displace soil.

- Earth limits water, as an earthen dam can stop a river.
- Water restricts or extinguishes fire.
- Fire controls or melts metal.

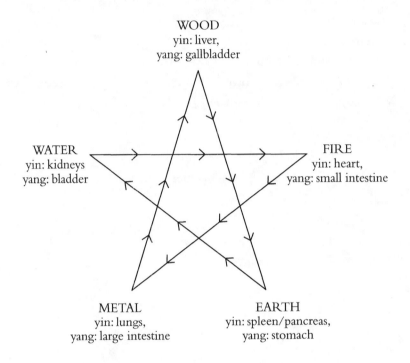

WOOD
yin: liver,
yang: gallbladder

WATER
yin: kidneys
yang: bladder

FIRE
yin: heart,
yang: small intestine

METAL
yin: lungs,
yang: large intestine

EARTH
yin: spleen/pancreas,
yang: stomach

The Controlling or Restrictive Energy Among the Five Elements
and their corresponding organs

Ancient Chinese herbal doctors applied this theory of the Five Elements to explain how our organs work in relation to one another within the whole. If you look at the chart on page 29, you will understand how the corresponding organs nurture and control one another in the same way that the Five Elements do. For example, the lungs, which correspond to metal, nurture the kidneys, which correspond to water. The lungs also have controlling energy around the liver, which corresponds to wood. We are at our healthiest when these relationships are in balance, and least healthy when they are out of balance.

THE FACIAL SENSES AND RELATED TISSUES

In their quest to understand how the body works, early scholars noticed many connections between the Five Elements and the five organ systems in the body. They also saw a connection between the face, organ systems, and tissues. They divided the face into five segments, or "senses," and the rest of the body into five related tissue groups, each corresponding to the Five Elements (see chart on page 29).

EYES, AND TENDONS, AND NAILS

The eyes reflect the condition of the wood organs—the liver and gallbladder. Sluggish liver function, for example, is often diagnosed by Western physicians when a patient has jaundiced or yellow eyes. The face may also take on a greenish cast if the gallbladder is out of balance. Chinese doctors noticed that these same patients also experienced extreme tiredness and nonspecific joint pain—indicative of tight, rigid tendons, or stagnant *chi*.

Deficiency of blood and energy in the liver will cause malnutrition of the tendons, which can result in numbness and tremors of the limbs. The Chinese also believe that the nails are the same substance as the tendons and require the same nutrients. Hard, strong nails indicate that the liver is healthy.

TONGUE AND VESSEL

Chinese legend says, "The tongue is the sprout of the heart." Thus the fire organs, especially the heart but also the small intestine, are linked to the tongue. When blood circulates freely and fully, the tongue—and the whole face—will be slightly flushed with a bright, healthy glow. Inefficient blood flow renders the face and tongue pale and white.

The tissue related to this facial sense is the *vessel*, a term used by Chinese physicians to describe the entire body. Without optimum heart and digestive function, the body is rendered out of balance. A Chinese doctor will use the color, shape, and condition of the tongue to diagnose illness.

MOUTH AND MUSCLES

The mouth itself is the facial sense linked to the earth organs. The strong, vigorous *chi* of the spleen encourages a healthy appetite, fully functioning taste buds, and rosy lips. The mouth is also the entrance to the stomach, the yang earth organ, carrying nourishment from the foods we eat into this primary digestive organ. This is how the facial senses, in this case the muscles of the body, are fed.

NOSE, SKIN, AND HAIR

Likewise, the nose is the facial sense that is related to the metal organs, particularly the lungs but also the large intestine. Strong respiratory function maintains circulation of fluids throughout the body, which makes for thorough and efficient elimination of wastes and activates defending *chi* energy. This protects the body by blocking the passage of airborne toxins through the skin's surface, while keeping skin moist and bright.

When the metal organs are "clean" and free of toxins, the skin and hair are radiantly healthy.

EARS AND BONE

The ears are the facial sense that relate to the water organs—the kidneys and bladder. The skeletal system, or bones, constitute, in this case, the related tissue. Thousands of years ago, Chinese scholars observed that if a person's kidneys, which they considered to be the basis of life, were not functioning, that person would die. In traditional Chinese medical philosophy, the kidneys are said to open into the ears, thus the energy meridian that links the two relates to hearing. When the kidneys are properly functioning and fully nourished, bone marrow production is enhanced, resulting in strong bones.

Other indicators of healthy kidney and bladder function are shining, healthy hair without grey, and strong, pearly teeth.

Traditional Chinese physicians often use these senses and related tissues as diagnostic tools. We will consider them as part of the total beauty-wellness picture.

NATURE'S SIX CLIMATIC EFFECTS: THE SEASONS

Here in the West, we see the changes in climate or weather as incidental to our health and well-being. The Chinese believe that these seasonal changes affect us deeply, because adverse conditions can disrupt our natural balance, both internally and externally, by penetrating the protective energy shield that envelops our bodies.

When we speak of "climate," we are talking about not only the external weather but our internal weather as well. Nature's Six Climatic Effects—wind, summer heat, dampness, dryness, cold, and fire—are associated with the progression of the seasons: wind with spring, heat with summer (which is different from the heat associated with fire), dampness with late summer, dryness with fall, cold with winter. Fire stands alone, both as one of the Five Elements (see page 15) and as one of the Six Climatic Effects.

These conditions can exist alone or in combination—wind-heat and heat-dampness, for example. When one or more climatic conditions are excessive, the body reacts in very specific ways, all of which can be corrected by consuming specific foods to nourish and balance the hot and cold energy in each system of the body.

Remembering the Organic Whole, we are part of nature. Our bodies respond to climate in much the same way as does the earth. Just as too much heat burns and cracks the earth's surface, excessive heat burns and cracks our skin and chaps our lips. Internally, the phenomenon occurs according to our lifestyle and the food we eat. Too much heat energy, caused by stress, anger, fear, or any degree of yang emotion, or caused by foods that are high in this same hot energy— deep-fried or spicy barbecued foods, for example—can disrupt digestion, causing constipation and even dry, cracked lips.

WIND

Chinese philosophy considers wind to be a climatic condition that is usually associated with spring but can occur any time of year. Wind moves quickly, just as pain and discomfort can move from place to place in the body. By its very nature, wind is often combined with other climatic conditions to attack our bodies—dampness and wind, heat and wind.

Wind is considered to be an external force. When wind attacks, it tends to break the barrier or energy shield of the skin and invade the upper torso. Symptoms of excess wind include head colds and flu-like symptoms. So, when the weatherman forecasts high winds, we need to stay indoors or dress in the appropriate clothing—scarves, hats, sunglasses—to protect our bodies from penetrating gusts. We also need to apply moisturizing creams to prevent the wind-caused dryness that chaps our skin and lips.

SUMMER HEAT

Although generally associated with summertime, excess heat can also occur in spring and fall. Although heat may be the opposite of cold, it too can cause chapped lips and skin. Oil production may be stimulated by summer heat, creating a variety of skin problems beyond sunburn. Perspiration and sebaceous oils combine with airborne pollution to clog up and enlarge pores. Make sure to clean your skin frequently and replenish lost fluids with creams or lotions that will draw moisture to the skin and hold it there. Drink plenty of water.

Excess internal hot energy results from too much yang *chi* in the gallbladder and kidneys, too much stress, as well as from eating foods that are deep-fried or too spicy. This condition can cause excess yang energy—fevers, boils, or flushed and blemished complexions. It can cause excess thirst, dryness of the lips and tongue, and, especially when the body has excess summer heat energy, strong-smelling urine due to toxins in the body. These toxins are the result of undigested foods and decaying waste in the intestinal and urinary systems. We tend to move more slowly during very hot weather and need to restore body fluids lost in perspiration by drinking plenty of cooling liquids, especially water, and eating foods that cool the body—melons, mint, tofu, green tea, cucumber, squashes, grapefruit, spinach, and tomatoes. The food chart on pages 46–47 will give you more suggestions for cooling-energy foods to incorporate into your diet.

DAMPNESS

The Chinese say that dampness is the prevailing energy of early fall, especially in humid climates. A little dampness—as in mild humidity—can actually be helpful, keeping the skin moist and soft. However, for some people, dampness can encourage germ and bacterial growth, which can result in skin that is prone to acne and other infections.

External dampness is caused by weather conditions such as rain, humidity, mist, dew, or even mildew and mold. Excessive dampness is sticky and lingering. Symptoms include rheumatism and arthritis, achiness, heaviness in the head and body, sluggishness in the arms and legs, bloating, cold sweats, fatigue, ennui, heavy secretions from the eyes and nose, diarrhea, and frequent urination or, conversely, water retention. The key to correcting these conditions is to cleanse waste and toxins from the system with special foods, teas, and topical treatments.

Internal dampness is usually caused by consuming too many cold foods—foods that are served cold as well as cold-energy foods—and by too much alcohol, coffee, and sugary drinks and foods (see the food chart on pages 46–47). As a result, certain functions of the spleen may be interrupted, causing severe stress on the adrenal glands. When the spleen fails to regulate the flow of fluids in the body, improper functioning of the elimination system results. It is essential that the body's wastes be expelled or these toxins will contaminate the entire body, causing colds and flu, irritated skin, and nonspecific joint pain—that creaky, achy pain you may feel before it rains. Pancreatic imbalance can lead to diabetes and other immune deficiencies and degenerative conditions.

DRYNESS

Dryness is most common in the fall, but can reveal itself as warm dryness in late summer through early fall and cool dryness in late fall through winter. It can also be created artificially any time of year, as in the warm dryness from a heater or furnace or the cool dryness from air conditioning.

Dryness, whether combined with cold or heat, is particularly damaging to the lungs. Internal and external dryness can cause dry, itchy skin, chapped lips, and constipation or hard, dry stools. External dryness can lower the body's resistance to illness by inhibiting its protective energy shield. This makes the body susceptible to illness and immune deficiency disorders.

Internal dryness can cause a decrease in body fluids. Such excessive dryness results in a dry mouth, nose, and throat; coughing, especially the dry, wheezy kind; constant thirst; cessation of sweat; and infrequent urination.

Restoring moisture to both the environment and especially the body is the best way to counteract dryness. If necessary, invest in a humidifier to restore moisture to the air distributed through your home heating and air-conditioning system. Take care that your body is hydrated inside and out. Moisturizing creams and lotions will ease dryness, itching, and flaking. To guarantee internal moisture, drink ten to twelve eight-ounce glasses of water per day and eat plenty of moisture-rich foods—melons, cucumbers, honey, avocado, sesame seeds, squashes, grapefruits, tomatoes, yogurt, and the like.

Also, stop smoking. Specifically damaging to the lungs and respiratory system, cigarette smoke invades the body's protective energy shield, lowering its resistance to healing.

COLD

Ordinarily associated with wintertime, cold conditions, like wind, can arise any time of year, especially once the sun has set in the evenings.

Everyone knows that when temperatures are very low, our bodies fight to maintain body heat. Pores close and capillaries contract. Blood rushes to the cheeks to help keep them warm. Cold can cause chapped lips and dry, flaky, or cracked skin. Prolonged exposure to frigid temperatures can even result in broken capillaries in unprotected areas. Although cold may initially stimulate blood flow and energy levels, after a while, energy levels may drop precipitously to conserve body heat, resulting in pale, even blue, skin. Protect your skin from external cold by wearing appropriate clothing and using protective lotions.

Symptoms of excessive internal cold can include loss of appetite, impeded digestion, joint pain or inflammatory arthritis, cold, pale hands and feet, forgetfulness, and fatigue. These conditions indicate an overall weakness or slow metabolism. While excessive internal cold is often caused by dietary imbalances, notably too many cold-energy foods, it can also be caused by long-term illness, surgery, or even pregnancy and childbirth. Warming tonics made from yang-energy herbs that generate internal heat— cloves, cinnamon, cardamom, ginger, anise and star anise, basil, rosemary, and sage—will provide relief. Refer to the food chart on pages 46–47 for more information.

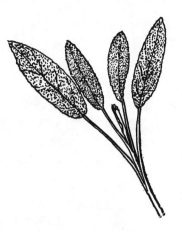

Sage (*Salvia officinalis*)

FIRE

The ultimate or extreme energy of all seasons, fire is both one of the Six Climatic Effects and one of the Five Elements. Chinese apply the term "fire" to *any* extreme or abnormal climate condition where symptoms associated with the original *chi* system are intensified.

Essentially, external fire is similar to heat, when the outside of your body burns up on a hot day. Internally, fire prevails when the body's *chi* is overstimulated or intensified. Smoking and exposure to smoky conditions cause "lung fire," while overeating or overindulgence in rich food and drink, with such symptoms as indigestion, heartburn, gas, and even ulcers, creates "stomach fire." Alcohol abuse and alcoholism create both "stomach fire" *and* "liver fire." Temper tantrums or frequent outbursts of anger cause "liver fire." Prolonged internal fire causes permanent damage to the affected yang organ–energy system and, ultimately, to the secondary yin organs.

Too much internal fire can cause fevers, flushing, bloodshot eyes, painful, swollen gums, and an irritated, bright red tongue, not to mention acne flare-ups. In women, the ultimate example of excessive internal fire is menstrual problems—painful ovulation, premenstrual pain, painful cramps, a heavy, dark flow, and irritability.

The only effective way to protect the body from the ravages of fire is to practice moderation in both diet and lifestyle. This includes maintaining balance in the systems of the body by nourishing it at a cellular level.

In the chapters ahead, I'll share with you some of the remedies—from foods to eat to formulas to apply topically—that are traditionally given to help balance climatic conditions.

THE FIVE EMOTIONS

While conditions caused by climatic conditions are, as a rule, external, those caused by the emotions are primarily internal. In the West, such ailments are considered psychological, or even imaginary, in nature. Chinese tradition states that five emotional states are at the root of many physical conditions. These emotions are anger, joy, sadness/grief, anxiety/worry, and fear. When these emotions are in balance, the body is stronger and has less illness.

The emotions cannot *cause* diseases but they can aggravate them, even injuring the health of the related organs (see chart on page 29). When the emotions are in harmony or balance, the body is without illness. When one or more emotions are too strong or too weak, physical symptoms may occur.

Western doctors are now beginning to accept the mind-body-spirit or emotional-physical link with illness. Physical ailments that are rooted in emotional conditions are no longer considered psychosomatic.

Problems arising from imbalances in the Five Emotions are more difficult to treat than those caused by climatic factors. After all, we experience a wide range of emotional highs and lows throughout the day. Situations arise, however, when an emotion becomes so powerful that it overwhelms a person's body and spirit.

ANGER

Anger has been found to relate to the liver, so too much anger can alter the flow of the liver *chi,* resulting in liver damage. To the Chinese, anger stems from an excess of heat (yang) energy in the bloodstream. Anger runs the gamut from resentment and outrage to jealousy and frustration. We believe that ruddy-complexioned people are more prone to emotional outbursts than those who are less "full-blooded."

An angry person often has a wide-eyed expression and tension in their joints and tendons—clenched fists, a squared jaw, and a taut stance. Left unchecked, anger can cause high blood pressure, headaches, dizziness, and even liver damage and gallbladder distress. The hot yang energy produced by anger and imbalance often shows up as acne in women before or during their menstrual cycles.

Repressed anger often results in stagnant or restricted flow of *chi* and, as with excessive anger, results in liver and gallbladder damage.

JOY

Everyone knows that happiness—joy—is good for the heart. This energy can give us a beautiful glow, but like everything in life, too much of *anything* is not good for you. An old Chinese proverb states that when one is excessively joyful, the spirit scatters and can no longer be stored. Excess joy is regarded not so much as happiness or contentment but as overexcitement or agitation. Too much joy can lead to "nervousness" or agitation and insomnia because joy is directly connected to the heart. It can also lead to intestinal upset, such as diarrhea. Too little joy exhibits itself in depression and oversleeping.

When joy is present, the facial sense—the tongue—is relaxed, moving with laughter; the related tissue, the body, or *vessel,* is in harmony.

ANXIETY/WORRY

Symptoms of anxiety range from moodiness and depression to obsessive and compulsive behavior. These emotions affect the spleen, pancreas, and stomach, altering the flow of the *chi* through these organs. The facial sense related to these earth emotions is the mouth, which in anxious times can be dry and tense, with lips pursed or downturned. Muscles, the related tissue, are often strained and tense.

According to the Chinese, too much anxiety can result in intense muscle fatigue, nausea, impaired digestion, and sometimes even in premature graying of the hair.

SADNESS/GRIEF

In the Chinese system, sadness and grief are associated with the lungs and large intestine. Sobbing, for example, originates deep within the lungs. These two emotions are generally treated the same way. Sadness and grief, when appropriately expressed in response to an incident or emotional stimulus, are regarded as healthy. However, when these emotions are overwhelming or unresolved, respiratory functions—the functioning of the lungs—can be disrupted. Anyone who has experienced intense sadness or has grieved for a loved one can attest to how this strong emotion can leave their insides in knots, proof of how the large intestine can be affected.

Tears of sadness and grief affect the facial sense associated with this emotion—the nose—by causing excess mucus, better known as a runny nose, and the related tissue, the skin, by causing redness, blotchiness, and sometimes break-outs. The hair, which is also a related tissue, may fall out in times of intense sadness.

FEAR

A little fear can be a good thing. It keeps us from stepping out into traffic or walking into dark alleys. In the Chinese tradition, fear affects the kidneys and bladder, interrupting the flow of *chi* in these organs. Chronic or unresolved fear—too much fear—can damage the kidneys or bladder and cause a variety of problems, from bedwetting and frequent urination to kidney stones, bladder infections, and in men, premature ejaculation.

In times of fear, hearing is intensified, connecting the facial sense, the ear, to this emotion. The tension caused by fear interrupts the development of bone marrow, linking the related tissue, bone, to fear.

Refer to the chart below, "The Chinese Way to View Your Body," for a clear picture of how the Five Elements are related to the body's five organ systems, facial senses, related tissues, and emotions. This intricate connection explains why your heart flutters with joy when you see your little daughter running into the room with a bunch of flowers, and why you may have an upset stomach when you're worried about those final exams you just finished. This also explains the connection between that red, runny nose you have when you've been crying, and why children sometimes wet their pants when they're frightened.

Problems arising from emotional imbalances are more difficult to treat than those caused by external, climatic factors. After all, we experience widely ranging emotional highs and lows throughout the day. Situations *can* arise when an emotion becomes so strong that it overwhelms a person's body and spirit. While hostile factors, including overwrought feelings, may cause disease, an individual's inherited energy system—*genetics*—must be considered. Other factors in this mix are lifestyle, relationships, work, diet, and exercise habits.

THE CHINESE WAY TO VIEW YOUR BODY

ELEMENT	YIN ORGANS	YANG ORGANS	FACIAL SENSES	RELATED TISSUE	EMOTION
Wood	Liver	Gallbladder	Eyes	Tendons/ Nails	Anger
Fire	Heart	Small Intestine	Tongue	Vessel (the body)	Joy
Earth	Spleen/ Pancreas	Stomach	Mouth	Muscles	Anxiety/ Worry
Metal	Lungs	Large Intestine	Nose	Skin/Hair	Sadness/ Grief
Water	Kidney	Bladder	Ears	Bones	Fear

2.

YOUR BEAUTY-WELLNESS TEST

ARE YOU PRIMARILY YIN, YANG, OR YIN/YANG?

Now that I've provided you with a wealth of new information about health and beauty in the Chinese tradition, it's time to discover how to put these principles to use. The first step in this process is to take my Beauty-Wellness Test to determine if you are primarily yin, yang, or yin/yang (balanced) in nature.

Don't try to look through the book for the "right" answers! There *are* no right answers. This test is designed to enable you to identify your current state of balance, or wellness. You will discover if you're primarily a yin type or if you are currently in a yang state. Some of you may even be surprised to learn that you are basically in balance!

Like *chi* and our cells, which are ever changing, yin and yang express the constantly evolving connection between body, mind, and spirit. Yin and yang are not absolute, exact conditions. We can be yin today and yang tomorrow. This test simply identifies your fundamental state.

BEAUTY-WELLNESS TEST

Select the most appropriate response to each of these questions and total your answers. This score will determine your primary state—yin, yang, or yin/yang (balanced)—so that you will be able to design the most effective program for yourself.

1. My age is:
   - 15 13 to 25
   - 10 26 to 45
   - 5   46 or older

2. My weight gain/loss pattern can best be described as:
   - 15 I can eat anything I want without gaining a pound
   - 10 Up and down, but no more than three to five pounds a month
   - 5   I gain weight easily

3. My appetite is:
   - 15 Hearty
   - 10 Moderate
   - 5   Light

4. My skin—especially my face—looks shiny or oily:
   - 15 Often
   - 10 Only in the "T Zone" around my forehead and nose
   - 5   Seldom
   - 0   Tends to be dry

5. My face breaks out:
   - 15 Often
   - 10 Occasionally
   - 5   Rarely, if ever

6. I have blackheads:
    - 15   A lot
    - 10   A few
    - 5   None

7. I have whiteheads:
    - 15   A lot
    - 10   A few
    - 5   None

8. I have dark circles around my eyes:
    - 15   Rarely, if ever
    - 10   Occasionally, during allergy season or when I am exceptionally tired
    - 10   Yes, due to family heritage
    - 5   Usually

9. I have wrinkles:
    - 15   None
    - 10   Only around my eyes
    - 10   Around my mouth *or* on my forehead
    - 5   Around my eyes, mouth, *and* forehead

10. My pores are:
    - 15   Large, open
    - 10   Medium
    - 5   Small, fine

11. The texture of my skin is:
    - 15   Coarse
    - 10   Average
    - 5   Smooth

12. I experience dry, flaky patches on my skin:
    - 15 Never
    - 10 Occasionally
    - 5 Often

13. I smoke cigarettes, and I would be considered:
    - 15 A heavy smoker (a pack or more per day)
    - 10 A moderate smoker (less than a pack a day)
    - 5 An occasional smoker/a nonsmoker

14. I drink alcoholic beverages:
    - 15 One or more drinks a day, usually every day
    - 10 Three to five drinks a week
    - 5 Occasionally/never

15. My hair is:
    - 15 Coarse and straight
    - 15 Coarse and curly
    - 10 Moderately thick
    - 5 Fine

16. My daily hair loss is:
    - 15 Very few
    - 10 Normal (80 to 100 hairs per day—there's hair in my brush but not an alarming amount)
    - 5 Heavy (I get a handful of hair when I run my fingers through it or my drain is full when I wash it)

17. My hair and scalp are usually:
    - 15 Oily
    - 10 Normal
    - 5 Dry

18. My fingernails are:
    15   Rosy
    5   Pale

19. The surface of my fingernails is:
    15   Smooth
    5   Ridged

20. I have sore throats:
    15   Often
    10   Once or twice a year
    5   Never

TOTAL SCORE: _____

YOUR YIN/YANG BEAUTY-WELLNESS PROFILE

IF YOU SCORED BETWEEN 100 AND 120 POINTS, YOU ARE PRIMARILY YIN

Yin bodies, like yin personalities, tend to be low-key, even cool, less emotional, and more reserved than their yang counterparts. If you scored primarily yin, you probably have a softer, rounder body than those who fit the yang profile. You often have dry, sensitive skin and a tendency toward premature fine lines and wrinkles, most often around your eyes and mouth. Your complexion and lips are often pale and you may suffer from the cold—especially in your hands and feet—not just during winter months.

To bring balance to your body, your diet should be full of warming yang-energy foods to increase circulation and rev up your sluggish system. These foods will not only lubricate your joints and internal organs but will also increase the elasticity of your skin. Yin personalities can have more hot, spicy, Jalapeño-peppered Mexican foods . . . and those peppery Chinese cuisines from Szechuan and Hunan! Add cinnamon, ginger, garlic, or dill to almost any recipe to give it the warm yang energy you need to achieve your maximum beauty-wellness potential.

One of my clients, Kitty, scored a solid 100 on her Beauty-Wellness Test. She fits the classic yin profile to a tee. Kitty, whose nickname stems from her catlike nature rather than her name, appears much younger than her thirty-two years. Only five feet, two inches tall, she has a soft, curvy figure and a soft, high-pitched voice—like Marilyn Monroe, the ultimate yin woman. Fair-skinned, with blue eyes and baby-fine blond hair that has the slightest bit of wave to it, Kitty is extremely sensitive to the cold, often complaining of cold hands and feet, especially during the winter months when, as she tells it, she goes into "hermit mode." Until she began to bring balance to her body, she frequently sought treatment from her dermatologist in hopes of finding relief from flaky, tender skin.

Kitty was so afraid of gaining weight, she eliminated *all* oils and fats from her diet. She refused to believe me when I told her that this contributed to her dry skin problems. The body needs fats for proper metabolism, and without them, it suffers. The results include flaking, dry skin, and low energy. Because digestion is slowed, weight loss is impaired.

IF YOU SCORED MORE THAN 220 POINTS, YOU ARE PRIMARILY YANG

If you could use only one word to describe a yang person, it would probably be "active." As a rule, yang types have lean, generally slender, body builds. If you scored primarily yang, you are probably youthful, outgoing, outspoken, and exuberant. You should not expect to age prematurely. Your hair and skin tend to be oily, and especially if your yang score is very high, you may be prone to acne.

The teas you drink and the foods you eat, as well as the herbal compounds you apply topically to your skin and hair, should be yin in nature to cool down or calm your fiery yang energy. Reach for foods that will calm your hot energy and bring moisture to the systems of your body, nourishing it and lubricating and toning your skin without increasing oil production. Choose yin foods— tomatoes, cucumbers, bananas, melons, citrus fruits, clams, crabmeat, and tofu. And don't forget green tea! That's the coolest of all teas.

Another spa client, Jan, is tall and slender with long, lean legs. At twenty-eight, she is the same weight as when she finished high school at seventeen. Headstrong, restless, and relentlessly independent, Jan dropped out of college her junior year to travel, which lead to a career as a travel photographer. Despite her active, athletic lifestyle and her health and fitness awareness, she thinks nothing of feasting on rare steak and spicy, greasy Mexican food. Her wild, thick, curly hair tends to be oily, as does her skin, which she abuses by too much unprotected time in the sun.

Before Jan altered her eating habits by adding more foods with cool energy to her diet, and treating both her hair and skin to cooling tonics and treatments, she had frequent and painful bouts of acne and intense bouts of PMS.

IF YOU SCORED BETWEEN 120 AND 220 POINTS, YOU ARE PRIMARILY YIN/YANG, OR BALANCED

Congratulations! If you fit this profile, either you were born with perfect original *chi,* or you are doing a terrific job on your own to maintain nutritional balance and are living a balanced life. Still, just because your yin and yang are in balance *today* doesn't mean they will be tomorrow! So your beauty-wellness assignment is to *maintain that balance.*

A person who has a yin/yang profile is generally even-tempered, alert, and fit. If you scored primarily yin/yang, your body type is probably neither too thin nor too fat; your skin is neither too dry nor too oily. By staying aware of your body's state of harmony, you will be able to maintain a high level of wellness and, as a result, optimum beauty. You will need to nourish your body with the right foods, and to lubricate, tone, and cleanse your skin thoroughly with the right topical treatments. You'll need to exercise to maintain muscle tone and keep *chi* flowing throughout your body.

Eat from all food groups; however, it is essential that you take equal amounts from each to stay in peak form. On pages 46–47, you will find a chart that lists foods by their inherent hot or cold energy properties. The middle, or neutral, column features a tasty list of foods that will leave you totally satisfied, including papayas, beef, potatoes, green mung beans, corn, chicken, eggs, pork, kidney beans, fava or broad beans, raw peanuts, and honey.

Another client, Margaret, might be described as "all-American Average"—

thirty-three years old, five feet five inches tall, brown hair, hazel eyes, with a fair complexion that turns pink before it tans. Except for slight breakouts around her period, her skin is decidedly normal, neither too oily nor too dry. Margaret has little difficulty maintaining equilibrium between her work and personal life. A moderate drinker, she laughs about being able to make a white wine spritzer last all night. She weighs a comfortable 130 pounds, and if she picks up a few extra pounds during the holidays, she can drop them in a month by leaving out bread and potatoes.

WHAT DOES THIS MEAN FOR YOU?

Armed with this information and with a greater awareness of the changes in your body, you will be able to adapt the special programs that are detailed in the chapters ahead to suit your body's needs. For example, in Chapter 4, I lay the foundation for your beauty-wellness program by learning the principles of detoxification, nutrition, and regeneration. In Chapter 5, you will choose from the foods and skin-care treatments—bath salts, scrubs, toners, and the like—that will soothe, moisturize, and tone your skin. In Chapter 6, I'll tell you how to care for your hair and scalp according to Chinese tradition and according to your type. You will be able to select the appropriate foods, soups, and teas to stimulate the systems of your body that relate to hair and scalp health while satisfying your tastebuds.

An important reminder: Be aware of your own physiology. By staying aware of your body's state from day to day, you can eat foods from *every* food group . . . in moderation. That's the key to balance.

3.

HOT AND COLD ENERGY— THE CHINESE WAY

FOODS AND HERBS AS FUEL FOR BEAUTY AND HEALTH

Everyone has heard that old saying, "Feed a cold and starve a fever." Or is it "Feed a fever and starve a cold"? If you adopt the Chinese health tradition, you'll never wonder again.

The foods we consume provide our bodies with nutrients that turn into thermal energy. So when you have a cold, it makes perfect sense to eat lots of special foods that provide warming energy to replace deficient heat in your system. Likewise, when you feel like you're burning up with a fever, eat cooling foods to extinguish that fire.

The Chinese practice is to provide our bodies with lots of cooling-energy liquids and foods to put out the fire—vegetables and fruits, plenty of water, teas and juices; rice or noodle soups that have plenty of clear broth. When fevered, our bodies almost always prefer yin or cooling-energy foods.

Just as health is beauty and beauty is health, the Tao of beauty acknowledges the ancient Chinese precept that food is medicine. However, we will not define the term "medicine" literally. We will look, instead, beyond the traditional

38

Western interpretation of medicine as having curative or healing powers to a purely Oriental concept that foods, as healing remedies, affect the health and wellness, and consequently the beauty, of the body.

This in no way precludes seeking the advice and treatment of a physician when you are ill. *The Tao of Beauty* teaches you to read the signals your body gives you. Perpetually cold hands and feet may be indicative of excessive yin or cool energy and a lack of yang or warm energy in your body. This condition may be resolved by eating foods that provide the body with additional yang energy, such as ginger, Chinese red dates, or dang quai. In the case of a fever and sore throat, your body is in an excessively yang or hot-energy state. The systems of the body can be brought back into harmony by rebalancing your body with yin foods—honeydew and watermelon, tofu, spinach, and cooling mint or green teas.

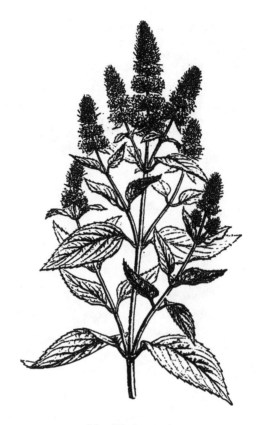

Mint (*Mentha spicata*)

I wish to make this clear again: The theories expressed in this book are in no way substitutes for your physician's care. However, with today's acceptance of more holistic ways of thinking, we know that we are ultimately responsible for our own health, and we can control aspects of it through nutrition.

THE HOT- AND COLD-ENERGY THEORY OF FOOD

By understanding the energy in the foods we eat, and how this can affect our well-being, we can optimize our vitality and consequently our beauty.

Remember, the energy I'm talking about is not only the kind that comes from the *calories* in food. That's a very Western concept. I'm talking about the *chi,* or life force, inherent in all things and how that energy affects the state of the body.

Everything in the world has yin and yang properties, but in this book I will concentrate on the yin (cold) and yang (hot) energy of foods. To avoid confusion we will use the terms *hot, warm, neutral, cool,* and *cold* when discussing the inherent energy in food—animal, vegetable, or mineral.

The energy quality refers to the basic properties of the food, not necessarily to the temperature at which the food is served. I think the best example is to compare mint, which is a yin or cold-energy food, and hot chili pepper, which is a yang or hot-energy food. The sensations inherent in these foods are easily felt. A cup of peppermint tea is classified as a cool-energy drink, even when it's served steaming hot. This is because mint cools any tissue it touches. This "cool" designation refers only to the energy inherent in the plant, not its temperature. A peppermint candy stimulates the same tastebuds as the hot peppermint tea, registering the same cool sensation in your mouth. Whether the candy is frozen, or (as is frequently the case) melted in the bottom of your purse, the effect it has on your system is the same: cool.

Similarly, hot chili peppers bring their hot energy and the sensation of heat into the body no matter how they are prepared. When you eat them, you feel their heat. They rev up your circulation and are hot enough to open the pores of your skin. Hot peppers make you sweat. This is a very efficient internal "air-conditioning" system for the human body, which is why hot peppers are frequently found in tropical climates. Lassitude and lack of appetite are common reactions to searing temperatures. If the weather is too hot, you simply don't want to eat. Mexican and Indian diets, for example, incorporate complex spice mixtures that not only cool the body but also stimulate the appetite. Spicy foods are commonly served with a neutral (or, as we say in our new vocabulary, balanced) grain such as rice.

As I mentioned in Chapter 1, our bodies, like our surroundings, are affected by climate. Our organs function best at the right balance of hot and cold energy, internally as well as externally. If we have a condition that indicates an excess of hot energy, such as a sore throat or acne-blemished skin, we need to consume more cool-energy foods to calm and cool the excess hot energy in our body. Or if we have cold-energy symptoms such as cold hands and feet, a runny nose, or pale, lifeless skin, we want to turn up the heat (or turn down the air conditioner), even though everyone else in the room is comfortable. We can resolve this by warming our bodies from the inside, heating up our organs with warm- and hot-energy foods and herbs. By bringing our body's internal energy to a warmer temperature, we can dispel the inner chill.

The following chart summarizes the basic properties of yin and yang energy:

YIN	YANG
Cooling	Warming
Relaxing	Stimulating
Deficiency	Excess

For example, eating cold-energy foods helps reduce excess heat in the body. This is helpful for people who have frequent sore throats, acne, and even constipation—conditions that are caused by excess hot energy. Typical cold or cool energy foods are:

- **Celery.** Drink celery juice or eat celery to clear internal hot energy. According to an ancient herbal medicine book, this is especially good for reducing excess heat in the liver and gallbladder and such symptoms as jaundice, PMS, anger, and dryness in the eyes.
- **Coconut Juice.** Coconut juice, especially from green coconuts picked before sunrise, helps cure acne and other skin rashes caused by excess heat in the lungs. It also relieves dry coughs.
- **Cucumber/Cucumber Juice.** Fresh cucumber and juice help cure common acne, caused by excess heat in the lungs and stomach as well as the spleen and large intestine. Cucumber helps detoxify the body by promoting urination.
- **Watermelon.** This summer gift from nature helps clear hot energy from the kidneys and bladder by promoting urination. This relieves edema and quenches thirst, helping to lower blood pressure and ease heat rash.

Foods that have hot or warming energy dispel cold energy throughout the body, stimulating circulation of both bodily fluids and *chi*. In general, hot energy foods help promote digestion and warm cold feet and hands, bringing color to pale skin and lips. A word of caution: Hot energy foods should be avoided by anyone with eye disease, inflammations, cough, or any other hot-energy symptoms. Typical hot energy foods are:

- **Cinnamon.** Heat a stick of cinnamon with a bit of sugar in apple juice or water, and sweeten with brown sugar. This popular winter drink is often served at ski resorts. Cinnamon promotes circulation through fingers and toes, warming limbs and easing rheumatic pain. It's also good for relieving heavy menstrual flow.
- **Ginger.** Used as a medicinal herb as well as a food herb by Chinese herbalists, ginger disperses cold throughout the body, relieves nausea, and stops motion sickness. It is also used to stop diarrhea, relieve asthma, and stop coughing.
- **Black or White Pepper.** Used to stimulate blood pressure and pulse, pepper is quick to warm the internal energy of the stomach and large intestines. It also stimulates the pulse and increases blood pressure.

ANATOMY OF A TRADITIONAL CHINESE DIET

The typical Chinese diet is very simple compared to the Western diet. It contains substantially more grains and pulses (dried beans and bean products like tofu)—40 to 60 percent in total. A traditional Western diet is hard-pressed to include 30 percent. The Chinese diet also includes 20 to 30 percent fruits and vegetables, with only 10 to 15 percent meat, poultry, seafood, fats, and dairy products. As you may have noticed from eating in Chinese restaurants, the Chinese eat little, if any, milk or cheese. We do enjoy eggs; however, we use them sparingly—one or two eggs stirred into a pot of soup large enough to feed the whole family.

Because it is neither too hot nor too cold, rice is considered to be the most nourishing grain. It is known to remove dampness, which is formed when body fluids fail to flow properly. Symptoms of this condition include fluid retention or bloating in the limbs and abdomen, heavy limbs, lethargy, poor concentration, and loss of focus. While other grains such as wheat, barley, oats, and rye are nutritious, they are considered damp forming. Consequently they are used less frequently, generally in noodles, porridges, soups, or stews.

Pulses—lentils, kidney beans, adzuki beans, chickpeas, green mung beans, soybeans and soy products such as tofu and tempeh—are considered cold or neutral foods. Because of this, they are most often balanced with warming foods such as ginger and garlic to assist the body in achieving optimum health.

Cooked vegetables and fruits cause less strain on the digestive system than raw vegetables and fruits. If you need to restore well-being to your body, eat these foods cooked. Raw foods facilitate elimination of body wastes and toxins, but can be irritating to the digestive system.

Meats, seafood, and the few dairy products found in a Chinese diet are considered highly nutritious. Because these animal foods have a potent concentration of nutrients, they should be eaten only in small amounts. A two-pound whole chicken will feed an entire Chinese family of six, whereas this little bird would barely make a meal for three in the West. This is because a Western meal most commonly includes a large serving of meat, a fresh salad, and some bread and butter or other form of processed grain.

The danger inherent in eating a meat-based diet, with more potatoes and processed grains and only a few cooked vegetables, is that your body is very likely to produce excess heat energy. This can result in irritability, aggression, inflammation, and weight gain.

Vegetarianism—the elimination of all animal foods and animal products from the diet is popular, especially with the monks. It is not generally recommended by Chinese tradition. Even a little bit of meat can be vital to your health, as the protein in meat helps form blood by nourishing the bone marrow. Blood deficiency, which is very different from anemia or a low red blood cell count, can lead to low energy, insomnia, anxiety, nervousness, brittle nails, thinning hair, menstrual cramps, and pale skin.

Following traditional Chinese nutritional principles, food choices are based on the energy needs of the body.

FOCUS ON FOOD ENERGY

Since ancient scholars developed the concept that all organs of the body are interrelated, Chinese health practitioners have studied how body functions can be restored to balance, and consequently health, by nutritional means. Ineffective treatments and formulas have been filtered out, leaving only those proven by time.

Drawing on centuries-old wisdom, passed on to me by my mother and other family members who have made this their life's work, I will introduce you to an amazing array of natural whole foods and herbs. You may be surprised to find that many are native to the western hemisphere and Western culture. Others are traditional Chinese plants that are generally available in the Asian markets that are flourishing in most large cities, large health food stores, and by mail order (see Resources, page 253). These foods and herbs will quickly become your primary means of providing your body with the nutrients necessary for health, wellness, and optimal beauty. In the Chinese tradition, herbs, especially, are essential to maintaining and restoring physical harmony while integrating *chi* throughout the body.

The food chart on pages 46–47 will give you an idea of the type of energy in foods that are commonly eaten in the West. This knowledge will make it possible for you to create a personal "diet" that is in keeping with *The Tao of Beauty* regimen.

Remember: Everyone is different. What is good for your friend is not necessarily good for you. If you scored a primarily yin or (cold) profile, focus on eating foods from the yang foods list to generate inner heat. This does not mean that you can't eat foods from the yin list. You can eat anything . . . in moderation.

Hot or cold energy can be neutralized by mixing them together, or intensified by adding spices, wine, or vinegar. Adding ginger or wine to any dish increases the hot energy. How food is cooked will change this energy as well. Stir-frying and deep-frying bring hot energy to a dish, whereas steaming has cooling properties.

If you scored primarily yin, you will want to design a diet that is high in yang energy to heat your inner *chi*. Drink ginger tea . . . stir-fry food with garlic and onions. Those of you who fit the primarily yang profile will want to increase your consumption of cool-energy foods to turn down that heat. Drink lots of apple or celery juice . . . eat plenty of melons. You'll also want to eat chicken or pork, which are neutral-energy foods, instead of beef, turkey, or lamb, which are warmer to enjoy the rewards of bringing your body into balance. Foods with balanced yin/yang (neutral) energy fit easily into the food plans for all profiles and enable you to serve a variety of foods suitable for everyone at your table.

This chart is merely a starting point, designed to give you an idea of the *chi* in many common foods. As you become more in tune with your body, you will begin to identify the conditions of excess yin or yang energy, as well as a yin/yang or balanced state, and you will gravitate toward the foods that will restore balance in the flow of *chi*.

COOKWARE ALERT

Whenever preparing, heating, or storing foods or topical products, it is recommended that you use glass, crockery, or enamel bowls, pots, and pans. To prevent interaction of the food with the metal, make sure that there are no cracks or chips in the enamel. This is important because the essential oils in many foods and herbs react adversely to metal. In a bath or topical preparation, this can merely render the special properties of the herbs useless or, at worst, irritate the skin. In a tea or food dish, this will nullify the effects of the ingredients and make the dish too bitter to consume. You could even become slightly ill.

For rapid stir-frying or cooking at lower temperatures, heavy stainless steel or some other nonreactive metal cookware can be used without risk.

Glass and/or enamel cookware, from saucepans to soup pots, can be purchased in any store for very little money.

WHAT YOU WILL NEED IN THE KITCHEN

I'm sure you already have most of what you'll need to prepare the recipes I'm offering in the chapters ahead. The only additional items you may want are assorted bottles to store my luscious bath salts and topical treatments.

You'll need:

2- or 3-cup glass measuring cup
8- to 12-ounce glass bottles with cork stoppers or tightly fitting lids

continued on page 48

THE ENERGY IN FOODS

YIN COLD/COOL ENERGY	YIN/YANG NEUTRAL ENERGY	YANG HOT/WARM ENERGY
Almonds	Abalone	Anise, star anise
Apples	Adzuki beans	Bell peppers (red or green)
Bamboo shoots	Apricots	Black pepper
Bananas	Asparagus	Brown sugar
Barley	Beef	Butter
Bean sprouts	Beets/beetroot	Cardamom
Black beans	Black fungus	Cashews
Broccoli	Black sesame seeds	Cheese
Carrots	Brown rice	Chestnuts
Cauliflower	Cherries	Cherries
Celery	Cabbage	Chicken liver
Chicory	Cauliflower	Chili peppers
Chinese cabbage	Chickpeas	Chocolate
Clams	Chicken	Cinnamon
Coconut milk and meat	Corn	Cloves
Crab	Crabapples	Coffee
Cucumbers	Eggs	Curry
Duck	Endive	Dates (Chinese red/black)
Egg whites	Fava beans (broad beans)	Dill
Eggplants	Figs	Egg yolk
Fennel	Grapes	Fried foods
Fish (white-fleshed fish)	Green mung beans	Garlic
Grapefruits	Ham	Ginger
Green tea	Honey	Guavas
Ham	Kidney beans	Herbs
Hops	Korean white ginseng	Jalapeño peppers

YIN COLD/COOL ENERGY	YIN/YANG NEUTRAL ENERGY	YANG HOT/WARM ENERGY
Kelp and other seaweed	Licorice (Chinese)	Lamb
Lettuce (all varieties)	Loquats	Leeks
Lotus leaves and roots	Milk (cow's milk)	Longans
Mint and peppermint	Oats/oatmeal	Mandarin orange peels
Melons (all kinds)	Olives/olive oil	(dried)
Mushrooms	Papayas	Nutmeg
Mussels	Peanuts (raw)	Onions/scallions
Oranges	Peas/snow peas	Orange peel, dried
Oysters	Pineapples	Peaches
Pears	Pinto beans	Peanut butter/oil/roasted
Plantain	Plums/sour plums	Pickles
Radishes, daikons	Pork	Raspberries
Rhubarb	Potatoes	Rosemary
Salt	Pumpkins	Sage
Sesame seeds	Raisins	Scallions
Soybean curd/tofu/milk/	Rice	Sesame seed oil
tempeh	Salmon	Sheep's milk
Spinach	Sea bass and trout	Siberian ginseng
Starfruit (carombola)	Seaweed	Sherry
Strawberries	Soybeans	Shrimp
Tangerines	Sugar	Smoked fish and other
Tomatoes	Tuna	meats
Turnips	Wheat and wheat germ	Turkey
Water chestnuts		Vinegar
Yams/sweet potatoes		Walnuts
Yogurt		Whiskey and wine

Bamboo steamer with lid

Blender or food processor

Bowls (glass or enamel), assorted sizes

Cheesecloth or sieve, for straining

Cutlery (sharp paring knife, butcher knife, and cleaver)

Glass or enamel saucepans, with lids

Mortar and pestle (optional, can be improvised)

Strainer (fine mesh)

Tea kettle (enamel)

Teapot (glass, pottery, ceramic, or earthenware)

Waterproof labels (to mark bottles of topical products)

Wok or large saucepan (stainless steel, not aluminum)

Wok utensils (spatula, strainer, cooking chopsticks)

Wooden spoons

COOKING WITH HERBS

The recipes I will share with you require little equipment and very little cooking skill. Before we get started, I'll give you some pointers to make preparation of these recipes even more of a snap.

Before you decide this is too complicated, let me assure you that most herbs can be purchased ready to use. How you use herbs will be determined first by the *form* of the herb:

- Leafy herbs, used fresh or dried, may be stirred into foods with little if any special preparation. Herb leaves should be muddled, or slightly crushed, before using: press them with the back of a wooden spoon against the sides of your bowl or cooking vessel. This releases the aromatic, flavorful oils into the recipe.
- For teas and many topical applications, you must prepare an infusion by pouring boiling water into a prewarmed glass or earthenware teapot or covered enamel or glass saucepan and adding the herbs. Cover and steep for at least twenty minutes to extract the energy of the herbs. Strain before using.

- Roots, stems, bark, and hard seeds require special handling. One technique is to make a decoction. Start by mashing the bark, chips, roots, or hard seeds with a mortar and pestle to soften the outer surface. Then put an ounce or more of the plant material into a glass or enamel pot with a lid. (Remember: the cookware should be nonreactive to the active properties in these ingredients.) Pour two or more cups of water, as specified by the recipe, over the herbs. Cover the pot and bring to a rolling boil. Stir once. Replace the lid and return to a boil. Reduce heat and simmer for ten to fifteen minutes. Remove from the heat and steep for an additional thirty minutes before using, for maximum benefits.
- Pulpy, fleshy roots and tubers, such as ginseng and dang quai must be steamed to release their inherent properties. To do this, put enough water in a saucepan to touch the bottom of the steamer when placed over the pan. Place the tuber or root into the steamer. Cover the steamer and bring the water to a boil. Reduce heat and simmer until the tuber or root is limp, approximately ten minutes, depending on thickness. Remove from the steamer and process according to the recipe directions.

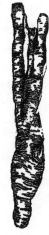

Dang quai

YOUR PERSONAL REGIMEN

Unlike traditionally structured Western-style beauty routines, *The Tao of Beauty* offers a regimen that fits your body's specific needs. You will begin by using cleansing tonics designed to remove waste and toxins from your body. The detoxification, digestion, and regeneration routines that I learned from my mother and other wise teachers are introduced in Chapter 4 and will start you on the path to natural health and beauty.

In the same way that you identified your primary energy profile by taking the Beauty-Wellness Test in Chapter 2, you will learn to identify what type of energy your body needs to restore its systems to balance. The recipes in this book will provide you with the kind of energy you specifically need. Note that I've indicated in the recipe titles which type of energy the recipe generates, yin, yang, or yin/yang (balanced). A recipe that is composed primarily of ingredients with cold or cooling energy will provide the body with calming yin *chi,* while a recipe that is made of fiery hot and warm-energy ingredients increases the yang *chi* in the body. Remember that how you prepare a food can alter its energy. An egg, for example, has neutral energy when boiled or poached, that is, when cooked without oil or butter. Once you scramble or fry an egg, it assumes yang properties. Another example: A raw peanut is neutral, but once turned into peanut butter it becomes yang in energy. In the same way, foods in combination can generate different energies than foods do separately. You need to bear all this in mind as you design a regimen that works for you.

Foods should be eaten in *balanced* proportions. *Nothing*—including steak and sugar—is bad for you, as long as it's eaten in moderation.

OPTIMIZING
YOUR
BEAUTY

4.

MAKING SENSE OF BEAUTY

THE BIG THREE: DETOXIFICATION, DIGESTION, AND REGENERATION

Now that you've determined your primary energy pattern—yin, yang, or balanced—and have been introduced to the concept of hot, warm, neutral, cool, and cold energy as it relates to our bodies and the foods we eat, it's time to put these principles into practice.

So, just as a painter must prime a canvas or prepare a wall before beginning work, we must make our bodies ready to accept the program of health and well-being that is the Tao of beauty. This is accomplished by three powerful processes:

- **Detoxification:** Thoroughly cleansing toxins from the body on an ongoing basis.
- **Digestion:** Cultivating eating habits that provide the entire body with the most potent nutrients possible, chosen and prepared to bring the body's into balance.
- **Regeneration:** Rest, relaxation, and sleep that empowers the body's

restorative powers to renew and recharge . . . a recycling program that makes it possible for our bodies to be nourished at a cellular level.

This healthy cell renewal process is as close as we will ever get to a real Fountain of Youth. It begins with detoxification.

DETOXIFICATION

What's the largest organ in your body? Not your heart, or your lungs, or even your liver. It is, in fact, your skin. All your mistakes in eating show up in your skin—from dry skin to oily breakouts.

The Tao of Beauty will teach you how to thoroughly cleanse your body from within—and keep yourself magnificently healthy in the process. You wouldn't put fresh makeup on a dirty face, would you? When your body is freed of toxins and residual wastes, every organ—every system—will be receptive to the nutrients and *chi* provided by the foods you eat. You will have provided your organs with a healthy, strong foundation upon which to build a healthy, beautiful body. Following the Chinese tradition, you must start with the most basic of functions to obtain the most rewarding results.

From the time we are born, toxins assault our bodies from external sources such as the environment and from internal sources such as extreme emotions and the wastes discharged by our organs. The body strives to cleanse itself of these toxins through the regular functions of bodily elimination: perspiration, urination, and defecation. Sometimes, if our bodies are overworked and have become weakened, we must augment these natural elimination processes.

Hundreds of years ago, Chinese beauties took special care to drink certain tonics—which we often call "soups" or teas—and eat certain foods only at specific times, usually according to the growing seasons of the plants used in these potent recipes. They learned that by drinking and eating in this fashion, they were able to increase their cell renewal while ridding their bodies more quickly of toxins and waste materials. Such poisons in the body can result in loss of energy, fluid retention, headaches, various skin conditions such as flaking, dryness, and acne, as well as other illnesses.

One of the most famous of the ancient tonic brews is called Four Seasons Soup. It is made of herbs for—and from—all four seasons of the calendar year. The formula is adapted to serve the body all year long as a basic tonic. Its ingredients are:

ANGELICA SINENSIS: Commonly known as dang quai, this root is considered to be the ultimate woman's tonic herb. It brings warm energy to the heart, liver, spleen, and kidneys. This is the primary herb in the fall tonic formula.

REHMANNIAE RADIX: This tuber is called by some "the kidney's own herb," as it promotes kidney function. It also cools the blood and counteracts dryness. In addition, it improves blood flow to the liver. This is the herb for winter.

LIGUSTICUM OR LIGUSTRUM: A highly aromatic herb with a bitter-pungent taste, this neutral-energy bark is most widely used to increase and improve circulation of both blood and *chi*. This is the herb for spring.

PAEONIA: Highly prized as a "woman's herb" this delicate root is said to purify the yin energy in the body. Traditionally, it is used to balance the female hormonal system and improve blood quality. This is the herb for summer.

Even modern Chinese women are known to prepare and drink this powerful tonic as the seasons change, altering the proportions according to the time of year. In the fall, for example, two ounces of dang quai are used, along with one ounce each of the other three herbs—*rehmanniae radix, ligusticum,* and *paeonia.* In winter, two ounces of *rehmanniae radix* are used with one ounce of each of the other three. The herbs are decocted—boiled—in four cups of water until the water is reduced to two cups. The resulting tonic is strained, sweetened with honey or flavored with cinnamon, and sipped—one cup the first morning, the second the next.

The ingredients, however exotic they may seem, are readily available at most Asian markets or Chinese herb shops. You can also mail-order them from the Resources listed on page 253. However, if you're not ready to take this step, there are numerous foods that you may already have in your kitchen or can easily find in your neighborhood grocery that will cleanse your body so that it becomes more beautiful from the inside out.

THE POWER OF TONICS

Regular use of tonics to increase organ function is part of both Chinese and Western traditions. In the West, however, cleansing has most often involved strong purgatives that force waste from the body. In practice, this can also lead to a depletion of the fluids, nutrients, and *chi* that your system needs, so you feel worse before you feel better.

In Chinese practice, the cleansing process is slower and is accomplished by systematic ingestion of herbal foods and tonics. Herbalists often give patients herbs to cleanse toxins from their bodies before beginning nutritional therapy. The complete herbal detoxification process takes from three to five days. Drastic detoxifying can be avoided by eating foods that keep the digestive system clean and clear on a regular basis.

The Chinese take tonics, teas, and soups not just when feeling ill, but as a regular, often daily, maintenance regime. Chinese tonic herbalism is the most basic program to promote optimal functioning of the body and to help the body heal itself.

Chinese tonics are herbal decoctions and infusions that work first to release toxins, then to provide the nutrients the body needs. In this way they strengthen the internal organs that require detoxification. As you can imagine, 5000 years of research has proved the efficacy of these formulations. Cleansing tonics, such as Chinese Licorice Root Tea on page 63, help remove toxins and waste from the organs of the body. Energizing tonics, like the Basic Ginseng Tea on page 62, stimulate the flow of *chi* through the body's meridians. For example, Chinese blood tonic does not treat anemia directly, as would traditional Western medicine, but it nurtures and stimulates blood *chi,* which encourages bone marrow production.

When I was growing up—even after we came to America—my mother made sure that the soups, foods, and teas that she fed to me and my sisters followed this traditional philosophy. Unlike American mothers who run to the corner drugstore for a bottle of aspirin or cough syrup when their children get sick, my mother went into the kitchen. And not only did she prepare delicious soups and formulas to make us well, she was also a great believer in regular doses of tonics to keep our bodies in balance. As dark as strong coffee, these herbal tonics were often foul smelling and horribly bitter tasting to us children. As soon as I spied my mother making one of her special medicinal tonics, I would often escape to a friend's house in hopes of avoiding a dose! Funny how that never worked.

As I grew older, I became more and more independent. Away from my mother's watchful eye, I ate out with my friends—fast food instead of her traditional Chinese fare. I was no longer the little traditional Chinese girl; I was now Helen Lee, a thoroughly modern American girl. The more I spread my wings, the further from the dietary traditions of my family I flew. I ate burgers and fries, pizza and sodas. I was just like all my American friends. I didn't think about the connection between my changed eating habits and the health problems I had begun to have—bouts of extreme fatigue and chronic acne. And like many American teenage girls, I wouldn't listen to my mother when she tried to tell me what to eat. I did not appreciate the benefits of my mother's tonics and special foods until I became an adult and turned to Mom for advice after Western doctors were unable to make me well.

HEALTHY KIDNEYS FOR A HEALTHY BODY

According to Chinese practice, maintaining healthy functioning of the kidneys and our other yin organs is integral to our health and well-being. Ancient Chinese healers found that a person's entire life cycle is linked to the condition and maintenance of the kidneys. Physicians observed that if a patient's kidneys failed to function properly, the patient would quickly weaken and die. Because these early doctors could only study and observe *living* patients—study of dead bodies was forbidden out of respect—this was amazing! These early scholars referred to the kidneys as the "root of life" and the "basis of life." The Chinese believe that the kidneys store the *chi,* the essence of life, and that they are the chief controllers of the reproductive system.

The majority of decoctions found in Chinese herbal texts are specifically designed to help the kidneys regulate their yin and yang energies. Together, the yin and yang of the kidneys supply energy to the twelve primary organs, thus controlling the basic *chi* of the body-mind at the cellular level. The kidneys are considered to be the body's most important organ-meridian system, since it provides power to all other organs.

THE HEALING POWER OF FOODS

In Chinese herbal lore, food is a vital healing force. Food and herbs are given the same respect and attention that chemical medicines are given in the West.

That is why so much of what Westerners perceive only as food is used in our most revered tonics. You may be quite surprised at what we consider detoxifying agents.

Detoxification rids the body of poisons and residual waste by promoting normal bowel function and regulating urination and perspiration. The simplest, not to mention gentlest, way to accomplish this is by eating a diet that is rich in detoxifying foods.

DETOXIFYING FOODS

Fruits and nuts: apples, apricots, cashews, coconuts, figs, grapefruits, ripe bananas, oranges, persimmons, peanuts, prunes, walnuts, watermelons.

Vegetables: adzuki beans, broccoli, cabbage, celery, Chinese cabbage, corn, cucumbers, eggplants, green beans, kidney beans, lentils, lettuce, parsnips, potatoes, shiitake mushrooms, snow peas, spinach, sweet potatoes, tomatoes, turnips, watercress, zucchini and other squashes.

Proteins: fish, pork, tempeh, tofu.

Grains and seeds: barley, black sesame seeds, brown rice, castor beans, oats, sunflower seeds, wild rice.

Miscellaneous: honey, milk, sesame oil, soy sauce, sweet basil.

FOODS TO AVOID

Beef and other red meat, Chinese parsley (coriander), coffee, crabapples, cured meats, fried and fatty foods, hawthorn fruits, processed or salty foods.

Please note that throughout the book many of the foods I suggest you try to avoid are considered nutritious and important to a balanced diet. I am not advising anyone never to consume these foods, only to use them sparingly. After all, moderation is the key to the Tao of beauty.

CONSTIPATION

One of the most important places to start in this program is with relieving constipation. Generally, constipation indicates that the body—especially the stomach and intestines—has excessive yang (hot) energy, a deficiency in *chi*, or inadequate moisture. The foods listed above help calm excess hot energy, increase *chi,* and provide moisture to organs; they are perfect for starting your detoxifying program. As I've said, you probably have many of these at home right now.

This natural Chinese detoxification process is considerably slower than its oft-used chemical counterparts, but I think you will find that it is decidedly less traumatic to your body. Although cathartic dosages of laxatives or enemas will purge the body of toxins, they can leave you with weakness and painful cramping.

As you begin to remove the toxin buildup in your body, drink plenty of liquids—water, juices, and soups—and eat purifying foods that reduce phlegm or mucus. Make time to include gentle aerobic exercise, such as walking, in your daily routine; this will also help strengthen your *chi.* I seriously recommend starting out every day with a long walk, followed by a relaxing hot bath. Walking helps to promote circulation of blood and other bodily fluids, and the internal movement of *chi.* The bath helps you to relax, and opens your pores to facilitate elimination of toxins.

I was born a yang, or hot-energy, type. Even as a child, I had major problems with elimination. By incorporating into my diet many of the foods listed above, my mother was able to restore the balance in my body so I could eliminate naturally. I also trained myself to have a bowel movement in the morning, when I am usually more relaxed, and established this as a habit I continued well into my adult life. This worked quite well until I became pregnant with my baby, Samantha. In my fifth month, when Samantha began to take up more space in my womb, she pressed against my intestines. Consequently, my constipation problems started again.

Thankfully, my mother reminded me of what had worked for me as a child. I was able to relieve this problem by drinking warm water with a teaspoon of honey on an empty stomach every morning for a few days. This helped to lubricate and hydrate my bowels. I also ate a special sweet-potato soup as a bedtime snack for a few days, and my constipation problems were no more.

Here are some natural laxatives that will encourage thorough elimination:

- In the morning, on an empty stomach, drink a glass of warm water with two teaspoons of honey stirred into it.

- In the morning, on an empty stomach, drink a glass of warm water with one teaspoon of salt dissolved in it.
- Drink a glass of warm water or green tea with one tablespoon of aloe vera juice stirred into it.
- Drink a glass of warm milk in the morning on an empty stomach.
- Every day, eat one or two ripe plums on an empty stomach. Other fruits that encourage natural bowel elimination are ripe figs, baked apples, and stewed prunes.

DIARRHEA

The opposite of constipation, diarrhea—frequent, loose bowel movements—is also evidence of toxins in the gastrointestinal tract. Possible causes are contaminated food and water, allergic reactions to food, infection by parasites, bacteria, or a virus, and emotional upset. These symptoms are often evidence of excess cool and are eased by nourishing the body with warming foods.

When diarrhea occurs naturally or while you are detoxifying your system, ease up on the cleansing tonics you may be using until symptoms pass.

- Avoid oils and fats, wheat foods, and milk products except yogurt. (The lactobacillus bacteria cultures in yogurt will replace the toxins that cause your problem.)
- Stick with clear warm liquids—especially clear broth or soups— for twenty-four hours. If you do not find relief, continue for one more day. Drink at least eight glasses of water a day to keep your body hydrated.
- Boil a half cup of brown or white rice in three cups of water for ten to fifteen minutes. Then strain, eat the rice and drink the water—one cup, three times a day.

URINATION AND PERSPIRATION

The body also expels toxins through urination and perspiration. Tonics and foods with diuretic properties promote urination and tone up the kidneys.

Foods with diaphoretic properties increase the body's internal heat and promote perspiration. A balanced diet, by Chinese standards, includes many foods with these properties. It is especially important that you have plenty of tonics and foods to promote urination and perspiration during detoxification.

- **Foods that promote urination:** asparagus, barley, black tea, Chinese cabbage, carrots, coconuts, coffee, corn, corn silk, cucumbers, kidney beans, lettuce, mandarin oranges, mangoes, melons of all types, mung beans, onions, pineapples, plums, star fruit.
- **Foods that increase kidney** *chi:* beef kidneys, black sesame seeds, string beans, sword beans, whole-grain wheat.
- **Foods that promote perspiration:** black pepper, black soybeans, cardamom seeds, chives, cloves, fennel, fresh or dried ginger, grapes, licorice root, lychees, nutmeg, peppers of all kinds, radishes.
- **Foods that warm the internal organs:** cayenne pepper, black or white peppercorns, chicken, chives, cloves, fennel seeds, dried ginger, bell peppers, lamb, nutmeg, green beans.

HOW LONG WILL IT TAKE?

Internal cleansing and detoxification is not an overnight process, certainly not after a lifetime of improper eating and elimination. I suggest that you start with one week of concentrated cleansing by following this program.

Black pepper (*Piper nigrum*)

- Every morning, drink a cleansing tonic tea, like Basic Ginseng Tea (page 62), Chinese Licorice Root Tea (page 63), or Wild Orchid Tea (page 64).

- Take a ten- to fifteen-minute walk at least once a day to stimulate the flow of throughout your body.
- Eat four to five meals per day, using any of the detoxifying foods listed on page 58, which stimulate circulation of, especially to the kidneys, liver, spleen, stomach, and intestinal tract.
- At bedtime every night, take a laxative tonic such as those suggested on page 65.

Follow this procedure for one week. Keep a journal of how you feel and how your body reacts to this new way of eating. At the end of the week, notice how you feel:

- Are you less bloated?
- Has your digestion improved?
- Is your breathing easier?
- Do you feel clearer and more focused?
- Is your appetite improved?
- Has your energy increased?

These are but a few of the changes you may experience as your body is cleansed. If you wish, repeat this detoxification regimen for a second week, then one week per month after that.

RECIPES FOR DETOXIFICATION

Basic Ginseng Tea   (yang)

Ginseng is the premier Chinese tonic herb. The Yellow Emperor's Classic of Internal Medicine *states, "Ginseng is a tonic to the five viscera, quieting the animal spirits, stabilizing the soul, preventing fear, expelling the vicious energies, brightening the eyes and improving vision, opening up the heart, benefiting the understanding, and if taken for some time, will invigorate the body and prolong life." Ginseng is an*

energy tonic, which replaces lost chi to the merid-
ians and organs. It is said to benefit the mind,
soul, and spirit as well as the body. This may ac-
count for its 2000-year popularity. For general
well-being, Basic Ginseng Tea, sweet-tasting be-
cause of the licorice and Chinese red dates, is
perfect for a detoxifying program.

Makes 2 servings

> 1-inch piece Korean ginseng (see NOTE)
> Two ¼-inch pieces Chinese licorice
>   root, cut in half (see NOTE)
> 4 Chinese red dates

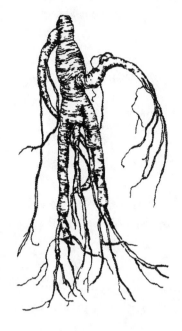

Ginseng root (*Panax quinquefolius*)

Bring 4 cups of water to a rolling boil in a
1-quart glass saucepan. Add ginseng,
licorice root, and red dates; reduce heat and
cover. Simmer over low heat for 1 hour,
adding water as necessary to retain 2-cup volume. Strain and drink.

NOTE: Available in Asian markets and health food stores, Korean ginseng is
the one most generally sold as "ginseng." It has a light tan to brown color
and is very hard. Korean ginseng has neutral energy, while Siberian red ginseng has hot yang energy and American ginseng has cooling yin energy. Use
Chinese licorice root only, available in Asian markets, health food stores, or
by mail order from the Resources listed on page 253. Its yang energy is a
powerful energizing and detoxifying agent.

Chinese Licorice Root Tea   (yin/yang)

In the Chinese pharmacopoeia, licorice root is almost as important as ginseng. It is
known as the Great Detoxifier because it removes toxins from the system and elimi-

nates any side effects from other herbs. In addition, it acts as a blood tonic because of its effect on the kidney and spleen—it brings chi to the blood. Served hot or cold, this tea has a wonderful taste. Chinese licorice has detoxifying properties that are not present in other varieties of licorice.

Makes 2 servings

> Four 1 x ¼-inch pieces Chinese licorice root (see NOTE)
> Honey to taste

Bring 4 cups of water to a boil in a 1-quart glass saucepan. Add licorice root, then lower the heat and simmer for 20 minutes, or until liquid is reduced by half. Strain, and sweeten with honey if desired.

NOTE: Chinese licorice root is available in Asian markets, health food stores, or by mail order from the Resources listed on page 253.

Wild Orchid Tea   (yin)

The Chinese orchid (Dendrobium hancockii) has been used traditionally in a daily tea to replenish the yin energy of the kidney. Suk Gok, as it is commonly known, is a sweet, pleasant-tasting brew that you will love serving to your friends. It's a perfect cool-energy tonic that prevents fatigue and replenishes the spirit.

Makes 2 servings

> ½ cup dried Chinese orchids (see NOTE)
> ½-inch slice Chinese licorice root (see NOTE)
> Honey to taste

Bring 4 cups of water to a rolling boil in a 1-quart glass saucepan. Add the herbs. Reduce heat to low and simmer for 20 minutes, or until liquid is reduced by half. Strain off herbs. Sweeten with honey if desired. Drink warm.

NOTE: Dried Chinese orchids and Chinese licorice root are both available at Asian markets and health food stores, or by mail order from the Resources listed on page 253.

Sweet-Potato Soup   (yin)

Sweet potatoes and honey are natural emollients, providing moisture to the gastrointestinal tract. This recipe is a natural, effective laxative and a tasty treat, good enough to serve as dessert, at the same time! This is the tonic my mother prepared for me to fight constipation.

Makes 2 servings

> 2 medium sweet potatoes, peeled and cut into 1-inch pieces
> 2 tablespoons honey

Cover the potatoes with 2 cups of water and bring to a boil. Reduce heat and simmer for approximately 30 minutes, or until potatoes are tender. Do not drain off the water, as it is good for you, too. Drizzle honey over the potatoes and toss to coat. Spoon the potatoes and broth into bowls. Eat at bedtime for 1 or 2 weeks as needed to relieve constipation.

Corn Soup   (yin/yang)

Here's a recipe that is a doubly effective detoxifier since corn also acts as a tonic to remove toxins in the stomach. It is also a diuretic, promoting urination and eliminating water retention. Chicken is an energy tonic that regulates the stomach and spleen. But that's not all: Eggs work as a blood tonic to help lubricate the stomach and other organs, including our skin.

Makes 4 to 5 appetizers or 3 to 4 main-dish servings

Seasoning Mix
1 tablespoon sesame oil
1 tablespoon soy sauce
3 tablespoons cornstarch
1 tablespoon sugar
½ teaspoon white pepper (optional)

2 chicken breasts, skinned and cut into bite-size pieces
2 medium ears of corn, or 6 ounces canned whole-kernel corn
3 tablespoons cooking oil
½ cup green peas
½-inch piece ginger, peeled and cut in half
2 cloves garlic, peeled and crushed
2 scallions, cut into small pieces
2 eggs
Salt and pepper to taste

Thoroughly mix the ingredients for the Seasoning Mix with 1 tablespoon water. Place chicken in the marinade and set aside.

Cut corn kernels from cob; set aside. If using canned corn, drain and set aside.

Preheat a 2-quart pot on medium-high heat until hot; add cooking oil and stir-fry corn, peas, ginger, and garlic for about a minute. Add 6 cups of water and bring to a boil. Lower heat to medium and simmer for 15 to 20 minutes. Add chicken with marinade and scallions to pot; return to a rolling boil. Reduce heat, and simmer for about 5 to 10 minutes, until chicken is cooked.

Remove soup from heat. Break eggs into a glass bowl and beat lightly with a fork. Pour into the hot soup, stirring once or twice to incorporate. Add salt and pepper to taste.

DIGESTION

I am often amazed that so many Westerners—especially Americans—accept indigestion, heartburn, and other digestion problems as normal. Just look at how many television commercials are for stomach medications and digestive aids. There are even pills that make it possible for you to drink milk and eat cheese and ice cream when your body rebels against dairy products!

There are many causes of indigestion, not the least being our obsession with thinness. Even young children who still have a lot of growing to do are dieting to lose weight. Constant dieting and irregular eating habits, from skipping breakfast and eating at irregular intervals, to anorexia and bulimia, disrupt the body's normal digestive processes. Such abuse can lead not only to stomach upset and loss of appetite but also to bloating, diarrhea, constipation, fatigue, and even skin problems. Consuming too much alcohol, caffeine, and greasy or spicy foods can lead to similar problems.

The concept of removing toxins and waste buildup from the gastrointestinal tract has already been discussed. However to obtain maximum benefit from this cleansing process and increase the absorption of nutrients by your body, it is vital that you bring balance to your digestive system.

According to Chinese tradition, tonics and foods that nourish the spleen are key to bringing balance to any digestion disorder because the spleen has a major influence over digestion and absorption of nutrients. The spleen is said to control the movement of nutritional substances and fluids throughout the body, and has a regulatory role over the entire gastrointestinal tract. It also influences fluid circulation and distribution, and works in tandem with the kidneys in regulating and controlling the amount of fluids in the body. Another function of the spleen is to regulate the quantity and quality of the blood.

Water is the best natural antidote to problems relating to digestion and the flow of fluids through the body. It cleanses and hydrates all of the body's organs, including the all-important intestines and skin. When I'm talking about water, I am referring only to water, with nothing in it. As soon as you put something into water, say, a slice of lemon or a spoonful of honey, this water becomes a carrier for the properties of the lemon or the honey. Such doctored liquids have an important place in maintaining the fluid levels of the body.

To illustrate the importance of good digestion, let me share an anecdote with you from my modeling days. One of the busiest times of year for many fashion models is early spring—March and April, especially. The rush starts in Paris with the couturier and *prêt-à-porter* (ready-to-wear) shows, then off to Milan, and back to New York. Models from all over the world make the circuit, working for as many as twenty designers a week. Between fittings and shows, there is little time to eat properly. Unlike New York and Hong Kong, where restaurants that serve nourishing food are open twenty-four hours a day, these European fashion capitals offered no such service. Restaurants in Paris even close between mealtimes!

One especially cold March in Paris, the shows were staged under a huge tent, which was so poorly heated that we were subject to dramatic temperature changes. Our days began at six or seven o'clock in the morning, when we assembled at the tent for makeup and hair in preparation for a nine A.M. show. After the day's shows, we would race off to rehearse the *next* day's shows. Often we didn't get back to our hotels until after midnight, long after room service and restaurants were closed.

Experienced models knew to carry dried nuts and fruits in their bags to keep hunger at bay. I was never far from my thermos of hot ginger tea, which helped to keep my body warm and my appetite up. I never feel like eating when I am particularly tired. One year, I shared my tea with my new roommate, Suzanne, who had mentioned that she was freezing. I gave her a cup of my ginger tea sweetened with honey, and she said later that it was one of the few times when she hadn't felt like fainting or that she was catching a cold. She also remarked that for the first time since she got to Paris her hands and feet were warm.

Suzanne confided that she often had digestion problems. Many days she did not feel like eating at all, and if she did eat, she had trouble getting the food down. She often hiccupped and belched, and once she threw up after a meal of iced coffee and a fruit cup.

We had a break in our schedules that day, so I took her to my favorite Chinese restaurant near the Place de la Concorde. Since I frequently ate there and the owners knew me, I asked the cook to add more garlic and ginger to our food. We had Hot and Sour Soup, Ginger Chicken, and Orange Beef, all warm-energy foods that are known to stimulate *chi* energy, increase circulation, and aid digestion. After this feast, Suzanne and I felt and looked so good for our next show that we barely needed blush on our cheeks.

The meal that we shared was just what the herbalist ordered! The foods and flavors brought hot energy to Suzanne's cold stomach and spleen and increased the downward movement of *chi* through her body.

THE POWER OF FOODS TO ENHANCE DIGESTION

Foods, prepared as tonics, teas, and meals, serve as aids to digestion in a variety of ways: calming nausea; stimulating appetite; inhibiting appetite; cleansing the digestive system; halting flatulence, constipation, or loose bowels; and promoting absorption of nutrients.

Whatever digestion problems you may have, the foods listed below will provide relief. In addition, they serve to restore balance to your digestive system—the stomach and the large and small intestines. For this reason, I recommend eating foods that provide the yin or yang *chi* needed to correct and prevent these problems. At the same time they will promote better digestion and nurture the skin, hair, and nails. Many of these foods are chosen for their own special properties. Papayas and pineapples, for example, are rich in enzymes that promote digestion and the flow of *chi*. Red and black dates, garlic, ginger, and sweet rice supply warming energy that strengthens the stomach's function.

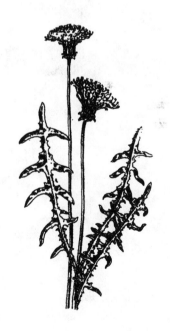

FOODS THAT AID DIGESTION

Fruits and nuts: apples, bananas, chestnuts, Chinese red or black dates, grapefruits, honeydew melons, kumquats, lemons, limes, loquats, olives, oranges, papayas, pears, pineapples, plums, prunes, star fruit (carambola), watermelons.

Dandelion (*Taraxacum officinale*)

Vegetables: adzuki beans, black beans, carrots, celery, Chinese cabbage (bok choy), Chinese parsley (coriander), chives, corn, dandelion flowers, fennel, lettuce, mung beans, potatoes, radishes, spinach, tomatoes, water chestnuts, scallions (white part), yams.

Proteins: chicken, fish, tofu.

Grains and seeds: barley, sweet rice, long- or short-grain white rice, oats.

Miscellaneous: black or green tea, brown sugar, cayenne pepper, cinnamon, clover, dried mandarin orange peel, garlic, ginger, ginseng, hops, milk, nutmeg, peppermint, sweet basil, vinegar, white and black pepper, wine.

FOODS TO AVOID

Alcohol; dairy products, especially ice cream; greasy and fatty foods; processed foods; red meat; all cold-energy foods.

WHERE TO BEGIN

You can relieve many digestion problems and ensure general digestive health by following these suggestions:

- Eat papaya—a whole small fruit or half a large one—twice a day after meals to promote digestion and to reduce gas and swelling of the stomach. Papaya also helps to relieve thirst and cough from fevers.
- Chew a few fennel seeds after a heavy meal to settle your stomach and dispel nausea.
- Fresh pineapple not only quenches thirst and promotes urination, which relieves water retention, but also has a balanced sweet and sour taste that provides neutral (yin/yang) energy that is extremely helpful in easing indigestion. Eat three to five slices or drink a four-ounce glass of fresh juice twice daily.
- Include tofu in your diet. It is nutritious and easy to digest, balances *chi* for general good health, and provides cooling energy that relieves the imbalances resulting from excess hot energy in the stomach and intestines. Like pasta, tofu is available in a variety of forms—soft, silky

soft, firm, hard, dry sheets, dry sticks, stewed, shredded. It requires no cooking, but can be cooked in countless ways. A good source of high-quality protein, tofu is also an excellent source of iron, phosphorous, and potassium. If it has been made with calcium sulfate, it is also a good source of calcium.

- Restore harmony to the stomach and expel gas by sipping a rice soup made with white rice and fennel bulb for breakfast. (See page 73 for recipe.)
- Spinach has amazing digestive properties. While raw spinach, especially, helps relieve constipation, cooked spinach brings cooling energy that extinguishes the yang *chi* that causes indigestion. Power-packed with the iron that a woman's body needs, cooked spinach also benefits liver function and balances blood pressure.

Incorporate the foods listed on page 69 to balance the *chi* in your gastro-intestinal tract, cooling excess yang *chi* or warming excess yin *chi* as required. The following are but a few of the tonics that are known to stimulate proper digestion.

RECIPES FOR IMPROVED DIGESTION

Mint Tea   (yin)

Mint is nature's own digestive marvel. Be it peppermint, spearmint, or simply mint from the garden, mint imparts a cooling, calming energy that improves digestion. Chew a sprig of fresh mint to freshen your breath and clear your palate. Brew an aromatic mint tea to calm a queasy stomach or improve a poor appetite. And for those of you who need to avoid caffeine, it's caffeine free.

Makes 4 servings

> 2 heaping teaspoons dried mint or ¼ cup fresh chopped mint, stems removed
> Honey to taste

Bring 4½ cups of water to a boil in a glass or enamel saucepan. If using dried mint, add the mint to the water, cover the pot, and turn off the heat. Steep for 5 minutes, or until desired strength, to draw out the maximum essence of the mint. If using fresh mint, muddle (bruise) the mint and add to the water. Simmer over very low heat for 5 minutes.

Strain tea into cup and sweeten with honey as desired.

Clove Tea (yang)

If you want to perk up someone's appetite, especially if he or she is recovering from an illness, brew a pot of clove tea. The warming energy of the cloves moves through the digestive system for almost immediate relief.

Makes 4 servings

> 1 to 2 heaping tablespoons whole cloves
> 2 teaspoons oolong or black tea of choice
> Honey to taste

Bring 4½ cups of water to a boil. Pour about ½ cup of the water into a porcelain or crockery teapot. Swirl it around to warm the pot, then discard. Crush the cloves slightly with a mortar and pestle to release the aromatic oils. Place cloves and tea leaves in the teapot and pour the remaining hot water over them. Let steep for 5 minutes, or until desired strength. Strain the tea into a cup and sweeten with honey as desired.

Tofu Spinach Soup (yin/yang)

Anyone who needs convincing that a vegetarian diet can be delicious should try this scrumptious soup. Spinach and onions are also proven promoters of digestive function, while ginger brings warming energy to counteract the coldness in the stomach that is the most common cause of indigestion.

Makes 4 appetizers or 2 main-dish servings.

Seasoning Mix
1 tablespoon sesame oil
1 tablespoon soy sauce
1 tablespoon cornstarch
1 tablespoon sugar

2 to 3 tablespoons cooking oil
2 to 4 scallions, chopped
1 small yellow onion, chopped
1 medium carrot, shredded
¼-inch slice ginger, coarsely chopped
2 cups fresh spinach, washed, dried, and cut into small pieces
8-ounce block firm tofu, pressed to remove excess water and cut into
    ½-inch cubes
Salt and pepper to taste

Combine ingredients for Seasoning Mix in a glass bowl and set aside.

Heat oil in a 2-quart enamel saucepan. Stir-fry the scallions, onion, carrot, and ginger for 2 minutes. Add 4 cups of water and bring to a boil. Add the spinach and tofu, and return to a boil.

Add the seasoning mixture, stirring gently to blend. Add salt and pepper to taste. Cover and return soup to a boil, then serve immediately.

Rice and Fennel Soup   (yin)

This traditional breakfast soup restores harmony to the entire digestive tract. It's also good for expelling the gas that causes stomach pain. The subtle licoricelike taste is a pleasant way to start the day.

Makes 2 servings

1 fennel bulb, coarsely chopped
½ cup rice

Bring 3 cups of water to a boil in a 1-quart saucepan. Add fennel and rice, and stir to mix. Cover pot and reduce heat. Cook for 30 minutes, or until most of water is absorbed and the rice is tender.

REGENERATION

It seems that in our busy lives, of all the things we truly should make time for and don't is sufficient sleep. One of our most basic functions, sleep is easily disturbed by the most minute of distractions. I can't emphasize enough that the Organic Whole—as described on page 9—must be properly nourished. So what does sleep have to do with nourishment?

Our bodies need time to regroup or recycle, to expel toxins, and to allow weary, overtaxed muscles and joints to regain their elasticity and flexibility. This can happen only when we sleep at regular intervals and for a sufficient amount of time. In clinical studies on sleep deprivation, scientists have found that lack of deep sleep not only impairs body function but can also cause forgetfulness and even hallucinations.

Without ample, quality sleep, you will not be merely cranky, your physical condition will suffer. Lack of sleep shows up in far more than dark circles and bags under the eyes. You may feel stressed and nervous or become prone to periods of excessive introspection, low blood pressure, or even fits of anger. Headaches and heartache are also common indicators that you are not getting enough sleep. Your hair may become limp and even start falling out; your skin may show the telltale signs of sagging, white- or blackheads, acne, or roughness and wrinkling, especially around the eyes.

WHERE TO BEGIN

Sleep must be approached as systematically as any other component of your health and beauty regime. The nighttime hours are the most precious time for your body's regeneration. It's best if you go to bed at approximately the same time every night and get up at approximately the same time every morning—

even on weekends. Sorry, I hate to take away the luxury of sleeping in, but it's true: There's no such thing as catching up on lost sleep. A regular sleep schedule helps maintain the balance of your system, and as you've probably gathered by now, balance equals health and health equals beauty.

Here are some ways to make sure you get plenty of the right kind of sleep:

- Make sure that the temperature in your bedroom is comfortable, neither too cool nor too warm, with enough ventilation for optimum breathing.
- Clean, sweet-smelling sheets are a pleasure we all deserve.
- Create an environment that is as stress-free as possible. The room should be quiet and dark, so that you can regenerate your body and spirit.
- Try sipping a calming tea—like Hops Tea on page 77 or chamomile tea—an hour before bedtime to ensure that sleep will occur naturally and quickly. You should not fall asleep like a rock the minute your head hits the pillow—that is a sign that you are overly tired and stressed and that your sleep will not be restful and regenerative. Ideally, your body should take five or ten minutes to dispel the day's stresses before falling to sleep.
- A warm bath—not too hot, or you'll be kept awake—will relax your muscles and your mind. I like to add a half cup of sea salt to relax my muscles and a dropperful of lavender oil for a fragrant, restful soak. Do this a half hour before bedtime.
- Onion vapor works wonders. Crush a small onion and keep it in a glass jar with a cap. Inhale the vapor just before crawling into bed. Most likely, you will be sound asleep within fifteen minutes.
- Deep- and slow breathing exercises can calm the most jagged nerves. Lie on your bed, flat on your back, with your arms at your sides, palms up. Close your eyes and begin breathing slowly and deeply, focusing your thoughts on positive, peaceful images—the sea, a mountaintop, or any other favorite peaceful place. Concentrate on the space between your eyebrows—your "third eye"—and mentally tell each part of your body, one at a time, to go to sleep. Start with your toes and work your way up. For other exercises to maintain the body's balance and help with rest and relaxation, see Chapter 10.

• Calcium, in the form of a glass of warm milk or tablets, prepares you for sleep and helps relieve muscle cramps.

FOODS TO HELP THE BODY REGENERATE

You may have to change a few habits if you are to have healthy, regenerative sleep, especially if you are accustomed to running at top speed from the moment you get up until you collapse into bed. The Chinese tradition regards sleep as only one component of total body care. Remember the Organic Whole, and approach sleep with the same reverence as you would your meals, exercise, and even work. You might begin by integrating into your diet some of the following foods known to support sleep—especially in the evening as bedtime nears.

FOODS THAT ENCOURAGE REGENERATION AND SLEEP

Fruits and nuts: apples, bananas, lemons, loquats, mulberries, papayas, pears, pineapples, plums, prunes, Chinese red and black dates.
Vegetables: adzuki beans, black beans, collards, fennel, leafy green vegetables (steamed or boiled, not raw), lettuce, mushrooms, spinach, white potatoes, yams or sweet potatoes.
Proteins: chicken, fish, tofu.
Grains and seeds: barley, brown rice, pasta, oats, rice noodles, sweet rice.
Miscellaneous: basil, chamomile, dill, garlic, ginseng, honey, hops, peppermint, rose hips.

FOODS TO AVOID

Alcohol; caffeine in coffee, cola drinks, tea, and chocolate; greasy or spicy foods; sugar.

Incorporate into your diet the foods that encourage sleep and stay away from the foods to avoid—especially those high in caffeine and sugar and those difficult to digest. These are sure to keep you awake at night, just as too much exercise near bedtime can keep you awake. When your body is trying to digest a heavy, fatty meal, the energy used to process this food—especially after a large evening meal—is bound to keep you awake.

RECIPES THAT ENCOURAGE SLEEP

Hops Tea   *(yin)*

Hops tea is a traditional Chinese bedtime sleep aid. Drink a cup or two of this tea every night before bedtime to relieve insomnia. It is also known to ease menstrual cramps, and taken a half hour before meals, cuts your appetite and eases cravings.

Makes 2 servings

> ½ cup dried hops (see NOTE)
> Honey to taste

Combine 4 cups of cold water and the hops in a large enamel saucepan with a lid. Bring to a boil, stir, and reduce heat to low. Cover and simmer for 20 minutes, or until reduced by half. Strain through a fine-meshed strainer and discard hops. Add honey to taste. Drink warm or cool.

NOTE: Dried hops are available in most large health food stores.

A-Date-with-Sleep Tea   *(yang)*

This relaxing bedtime drink is also great for those with weak stomachs. Red dates contain warming energy and act as a tonic for the spleen, stomach, and blood. Red dates are naturally sweet, therefore no other sweetener is needed.

Makes 1 serving

> 5 Chinese red dates, pitted (see NOTE)
> 4 scallions, white part only, peeled

Combine the dates and scallions with 1½ cups of water in an enamel or glass saucepan, and bring to a boil. Reduce temperature to medium and

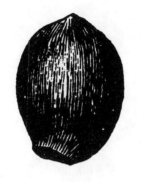

Chinese red date (*Cycas revoluta*)

simmer until reduced to 1 cup. Strain before drinking, but you can eat the dates and scallion heads if desired.

NOTE: Chinese red dates are available in Asian grocery stores, herbal shops, many large health food stores, or by mail order from the Resources listed on page 253.

Wheat and Red Date Soup (yin/yang)

The cool energy of the wheat counteracts the hot energy of the dates and promotes optimum heart, spleen, and kidney function. Wheat is traditionally used in Chinese medicine to help calm those who are prone to emotional upsets.

Makes 1 serving

> 1 teaspoon wheat germ
> 4 to 6 pitted Chinese red dates (see NOTE)
> 1-inch piece Chinese licorice root (see NOTE)

Toast the wheat germ in a dry skillet without oil until it is a light golden color. Cover the wheat and red dates with 1½ cups water in a glass or enamel saucepan. Bring to a boil and reduce heat. Add licorice root and simmer over medium heat until the water is reduced to 1 cup. Strain. Drink the tea and eat the red dates for restful sleep.

NOTE: Be sure to use Chinese licorice root; it has properties not found in other varieties. Chinese red dates and Chinese licorice root are both available in Asian markets, health food stores, or by mail order from the Resources listed on page 253.

Siren-of-the-Sea Bath Salts   *(yin)*

This is not a recipe to eat, but one to luxuriate in. The cool energy of the miraculous marine plants draws toxins from your body and cleanses your skin while completely relaxing your body. Pour these salts into your bedtime bath, and the glorious scent of the ocean is yours.

Makes 16 ounces, enough for 3 to 4 baths

¼ cup kombu (see NOTE)
¼ cup dulse (see NOTE)
2 cups coarse-ground sea salt
½ cup liquid soap (see NOTE)
1 tablespoon light oil (canola, almond, avocado, olive)

Pulverize the dried kombu and dulse in a blender, then pour into a large glass bowl. Add sea salt and stir until it is thoroughly incorporated. Add the liquid soap and the oil. Stir well, until mixture resembles lumpy oatmeal.

Pour the salt mixture onto a clean flat surface such as a cookie sheet, and store overnight, uncovered, in a warm, dry place. Stir to make certain mixture is dry. If not, place in a 200°F oven and bake for 15 minutes only. Do not microwave. Pour into a clean, airtight container—preferably glass.

NOTE: Kombu and dulse are seaweeds, sold in health food stores, macrobiotic food stores, and Asian markets. For liquid soup, try Dr. Bronner's Unscented Baby Castile Soap, which is widely available in drugstores and health food stores.

5.

TAKING CARE OF YOUR SKIN

THE CHINESE TOUCH FOR HEALTHY, RADIANT SKIN

Highly prized in all cultures, beautiful skin is a sign of youth, health, and vitality. According to traditional Chinese practice, this crucial aspect of your appearance can be attained by combining external regimens with internal ones.

In China, glowing, toned skin is regarded as a prime indicator of overall good health, strong circulation, and good *chi*. In contrast, here in the West we focus on what we put *on* our faces, not what we put *in* our bodies. As a result, no matter how expensive the lotion, it is bound to fail, for nothing can replace the inner glow that comes from abundant health.

Diet is the key component of the Tao of beauty. The food you eat has *everything* to do with the way you look. Some foods improve the condition of your skin enormously; others can harm it when eaten in excess. As you know from Chapter 4, poor digestion, constipation, erratic sleeping habits, and unsettled emotions, not to mention external issues such as air pollution, can take their toll on your body and consequently your beauty. How then, with all this assault, can you reclaim the youthful appearance you desire? It's easier than you think, once you accept the dictum that balance is everything.

The concepts of hot and cold energy in foods and how their respective yin or yang qualities (alone and synergistically) can affect us have already been introduced. Understanding your own beauty-wellness profile from Chapter 2 and learning how to achieve the best possible balance for your ever-changing body chemistry are key to achieving the skin you seek. Cosmetics and topical applications are helpful, to be sure, but the place to start is with your diet.

A DIFFERENT APPROACH

When clients come into my salon, they are surprised that I spend more time discussing what they eat than I do telling them about skin care and cosmetics. As you wouldn't put makeup on a dirty face, you cannot cover up a lifetime of bad eating habits. This is a radically different concept from what is generally taught in the West, but believe me, it's true.

Sandra is the perfect example. Tall and slender, she could have been quite beautiful except for the rampant acne that no amount of foundation could disguise. She sauntered into my salon with an obvious chip on her shoulder. Before I could even say hello, she snapped, "Give me something for my skin. I don't care what it is, I know it won't work anyway."

As I asked her questions, I began to understand her cynical attitude. Plagued with acne since she was a teenager, she had gone from salon to salon and dermatologist to dermatologist for years. No matter how much money she spent, nothing had worked. She was now a successful lawyer, and she felt her blemished skin was detracting from her work performance.

I understood how she felt and started immediately to analyze her problem, which was certainly more than skin deep. Her *chi,* which was primarily hot, was seriously out of balance.

First, I asked what she used to wash her face. Just as I suspected, she was using a commercial cleanser with far too much oil for her skin type. As a result, her face was never really getting clean. The lingering dead skin cells blocked her pores, exacerbating ingrown facial hairs that she had to tweeze to remove.

Sandra told me that she had dry skin, and the surface was certainly patchy and parched. But I explained to her that the dehydrated skin was actually layers of dead cells that adhered to the skin's surface because of its excess *oiliness*. She had been using astringent products in an attempt to *stop* oiliness and, as a result, had stimulated oil production. I started her on a regimen of balanced skin-care products that would correct this—including a gentle ginseng-mint cleanser, the Chamomile-Mint Toner on page 92 and the Honey-Lemon Moisturizing Treatment on page 93. I also recommended that she use the Chrysanthemum-Chamomile Mask (page 93) to deep-clean her oily—rather than dry, as she had thought—skin. This would dissipate the heat of her blemishes and promote the natural exfoliation and renewal of her complexion.

Under this new regimen of skin care and diet, Sandra's skin showed improvement almost immediately and cleared up completely within a few weeks. It's stayed that way, too. More importantly, her yin and yang energies were back in balance—she was relaxed and happy!

THE POWER OF FOODS TO IMPROVE SKIN

While most beauty books deal only with the surface of the skin, *The Tao of Beauty* starts with the *chi* energy of your body. The only way to keep this flowing without interruption is by nourishing every organ in the body. In this chapter, I'll discuss the organ that affects beauty the most—the skin. The most important elements of beautiful skin are proper diet, elimination, rest, and topical skin care.

The foods listed below are known to nourish the organs of the body that influence the condition of the skin, particularly the lungs and large intestine. As I explained in Chapter 1, the skin is the tissue related to these organs. The skin is the body's largest organ, key to the elimination of toxins and body waste through perspiration, the heart and circulatory system, as well as the entire digestive tract. Be aware that some foods can be helpful in treating one skin condition but irritating to another. For example, pineapple, which restores moisture to the body, hydrating dry, rough skin, is too acidic for anyone with acne. You'll find more specific food recommendations in the explanation of care for each skin type.

FOODS THAT PROMOTE HEALTHY SKIN

Fruits and nuts: Asian pears, bananas, blackberries, cherries, crabapples, lemons, melons, papayas, plums, Chinese red and black dates.

Vegetables: adzuki beans, avocados, bean sprouts, broccoli and other dark green vegetables, carrots, celery, chickpeas, chicory, cucumbers, dandelion flowers, garlic, ginger, green beans, leeks, lentils, black beans, mung beans, onions, pumpkins, radishes, seaweed (especially arame, hijiki, and kelp), spinach, sweet potatoes, water chestnuts, watercress, winter squashes.

Grains and seeds: black sesame seeds, brown rice, millet, sunflower seeds, whole grains.

Proteins: chicken, clams, fish (especially low-fat white fish such as cod, haddock, flounder and scrod).

Miscellaneous: cinnamon bark, goldenseal, honey, honeysuckle, licorice root, mint, nettles, peppermint, red clover, safflower oil, sharkfin, wood ear fungus, all foods with high collagen.

FOODS TO AVOID

Alcoholic and carbonated beverages, caffeine, canned and refined foods (including tuna), cheese and other dairy products, eggs, fatty foods, nut butters, red meat, sugary foods and drinks, white flour, white pasta.

THE TAO OF BEAUTY SKIN-CARE PROGRAM

The following chart outlines the suggested beauty regimen for your skin type or condition. I've included recipes for these topical treatments as well as for nourishing foods and teas that will bring health and balance to your skin. Include as many of these foods as possible into your diet. They are listed above and in the sections that discuss specific skin conditions.

Cleansers and scrubs, toners, moisturizers, masks, and baths are to be used as needed, some daily or weekly, as part of your regular skin-care routine, or as indicated by the condition of your skin.

THE TAO OF BEAUTY SKIN-CARE PROGRAM

	CLEANSERS AND SCRUBS *Use Daily*	TONERS AND SPLASHES *Use Daily*	MOISTURIZERS *Use as Needed*	SPECIAL MASKS *Use Weekly*	TREATMENTS *Use as Needed*
Normal Skin	Walnut–Yogurt Scrub *Page 87*	Chrysanthemum Mint Toner *Page 87*	Ginseng–Mayo Moisturizer *Page 88*	Honey–Apricot Mask *Page 89*	Warm Wine Bath *Page 89*
Oily Skin	Barley–Strawberry Yogurt Scrub *Page 92*	Chamomile-Mint Toner *Page 92*	Honey–Lemon Moisturizer *Page 93*	Chrysanthemum-Chamomile Mask *Page 93*	
Acne	Barley-Lime-Honey Cleanser *Page 96*	Sunset Citrus Splash *Page 97*	Lavender-Aloe Moisturizer *Page 97*	Mint-Clay Mask *Page 98*	
Dry Skin	Oatmeal-Honey Scrub *Page 100*	Slippery Elm Splash *Page 101*	Ginseng-Almond Luxury Lotion *Page 101*	Morning Star Detoxifying Mask *Page 102*	
Combo Skin	Honey-Mint-Barley Scrub *Page 104*	Parsley Toner *Page 104*	Raw-Honey Moisturizer *Page 105*	Bay Leaf and Clay Mask *Page 105*	
Sensitive or Allergic Skin	Egg White and Honey Cleanser *Page 108*	Comfrey-Raspberry Splash *Page 109*	Honey-Avocado Body Moisturizer *Page 109*	Clay-Milk Mask *Page 110*	Honeysuckle Skin Steam *Page 110*
Eczema	Papaya-Yogurt Body Scrub *Page 114*	Thyme-Lavender Toner *Page 114*	Chamomile-Aloe Moisturizer *Page 115*	Comfrey, Honey, and Egg Mask *Page 115*	
Liver Spots	Papaya Bleaching Scrub *Page 117*	Eucalyptus–Witch Hazel–Lemon Toner *Page 117*	Happy Honeysuckle Oil *Page 118*	Supersweet Spot-Removing Mask *Page 119*	
Sun-Damaged Skin	Oatmeal Water–Vinegar Wash *Page 120*	Lettuce–Water Splash *Page 121*	Aloe–Green Tea Moisturizer *Page 121*	Honey-Aloe Mask *Page 122*	Dang Quai Damage Control Cream Mandarin Miracle Body Cream *Page 122, 123*

IF YOU HAVE NORMAL (BALANCED) SKIN

One of the signs of a wonderful energy balance is normal skin—skin that is neither too dry nor too oily, too sensitive, nor too rough.

The main thing to remember is that although you may be balanced today, tomorrow your skin may erupt or get a bit dry. You may notice that when you are menstruating, your skin breaks out a bit, or if you're upset or under stress at work, your skin may become dry. Your task is to avert skin problems by maintaining balanced *chi* throughout your body.

Betsy, a nurse in her forties, told me that she maintains her beautifully balanced complexion by eating a balanced diet and having weekly facials, which include the Honey-Apricot Mask on page 89. She doesn't smoke, and she stays out of smoky environments as much as possible. Betsy never sunbathes, and also uses sunscreen whenever she's outside, regardless of the time of year.

Hostile factors in our environment—pollution, for example—and overwrought emotions are not the only causes of problems for normal skin. Chinese medicine recognizes that an individual's inherited energy system (genetics) plays a large part in determining how we handle the many distresses in our lives. Your lifestyle and work, exercise, and diet all play a part in maintaining health and beauty. Of these, Chinese experts consider diet to be the most important.

Although the following recipes are designed to maintain the balance of normal skin, they can be used by anyone, regardless of skin type or condition.

RECIPES FOR NORMAL SKIN

Salmon-Asparagus Stir-Fry   (yin/yang)

Neutral foods—like salmon and asparagus—star in this beautifully balanced entrée. Asparagus, as well as the almonds that garnish this delicate dish, are known to moisturize lung tissue, which improves skin quality and helps you maintain a dewy, youthful look.

Makes 2 to 4 main-dish servings

Seasoning Mix
¼ cup soy sauce
½ cup white wine, rice wine, or sherry
1 teaspoon sugar

1 pound salmon steak, 1 inch thick, cut into ½-inch strips (see NOTE)
4 to 6 cloves garlic, coarsely chopped
6 to 8 scallions, cut into 1-inch pieces
1½-inch piece ginger, peeled and sliced into 6 to 8 pieces
1 or 2 dried red chili peppers, seeds and membranes removed (optional)
3 to 4 tablespoons cooking oil
1 bunch (about 1 pound) thin asparagus spears, ends removed and cut
    into 1-inch pieces
½ cup toasted almond slivers, for garnish

Combine Seasoning Mix ingredients in a large glass bowl. Add the salmon and toss gently to coat. Cover bowl with plastic wrap and marinate 15 minutes.

Divide garlic, scallions, ginger, and pepper into two equal portions. Drain the fish and reserve half of the marinade (discard the other half).

Heat oil in a wok or iron skillet over medium heat. Add half of the garlic, scallions, ginger, and pepper and stir quickly to release flavors. Add the drained fish and stir-fry over high heat for 2 to 3 minutes, until about half done. Add remaining garlic, scallions, ginger, and pepper, and asparagus; stir-fry for 3 minutes. Add the reserved marinade; reduce heat to low and simmer 2 to 3 minutes, until fish and asparagus are cooked.

Garnish with almond slivers. Serve over rice, if desired.

NOTE: You can use tuna or any other lean, thick fish; boneless chicken breasts; or, for vegetarians, firm tofu with excess water pressed out.

Walnut-Yogurt Scrub   (yin/yang)

Chinese women traditionally eat walnuts with rice as a breakfast "beauty food." Walnuts are high in nutritious oils similar to the body's natural oils, which lubricate without clogging the skin. When applied topically, walnuts have the same effect without the extra calories. Yogurt is great for maintaining the body's natural acid mantle, which combats the free radicals that age your skin.

Makes 1 treatment

   ¼ cup finely chopped walnuts
   ¼ cup plain yogurt

In a blender mix the walnuts thoroughly with the yogurt. Wet your face, then rub gently into your skin to cleanse and exfoliate, taking care to avoid the delicate tissue around your eyes. Rinse off with tepid water and pat face dry with a soft towel.

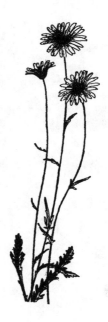

Chrysanthemum
(*Chrisantemum
leucanthemum*)

Chrysanthemum-Mint Toner   (yin/yang)

Chrysanthemum flowers and mint, taken internally, help the body withstand heat. Applied externally, they cool any hot energy in the skin and maintain balance in your body. The remaining ingredients in this special toning lotion help to exfoliate dead cells and bring life to your complexion. You can even drink this as a tea with just the smallest touch of honey.

Makes 7 to 10 applications

   1 tablespoon dried chrysanthemum petals (see NOTE)
   1 tablespoon dried chamomile flowers (see NOTE)

1 tablespoon dried mint
1 tablespoon buckwheat
1 tablespoon lemon juice

Bring 2 cups of water to a boil in a medium-sized glass or enamel saucepan. Reduce heat and add all the herbs and buckwheat, then simmer for 30 minutes. Cool; strain mixture through a sieve and discard herbs. Add lemon juice to the liquid and stir to mix.

To use, pour 1 to 2 tablespoons into a glass bowl and apply to the face with cotton balls once or twice a day (do not use directly from bottle to prevent contamination). Store in a tightly closed glass container in refrigerator for up to 1 week.

NOTE: Dried chrysanthemum petals and dried chamomile are available in herb shops and health foods stores or by mail order from the Resources listed on page 253.

Ginseng-Mayo Moisturizer   (yin/yang)

This moisturizing mixture is truly a meeting of East and West. Ginseng has properties that maintain the skin's natural acid mantle, while the eggs and oil in the mayonnaise act as humectants to attract water into the cells.

Makes 1 treatment

2 tablespoons ginseng powder (see NOTE)
4 tablespoons mayonnaise

Mix the ginseng powder with the mayonnaise in a small bowl or cup, stirring thoroughly. Apply to your freshly scrubbed face; let sit for 5 minutes, then wash off. Pat face dry with a soft towel.

NOTE: Ginseng powder is available in Asian markets and health food stores.

Honey-Apricot Mask   (yin/yang)

For those with normal or balanced skin, here's a marvelous neutral mask that will hydrate and soften your skin at the same time. It's not just for your face! Use it all over your body for soft, glowing skin.

Makes 1 facial or body treatment

> ½ cup honey
> 2 apricots, peeled and coarsely chopped

Measure honey into a glass bowl. Add the apricots and mix together with a wooden spoon. Apply to your face and neck, massaging gently with your fingertips. Leave on 10 minutes. Rinse off with tepid water. Pat skin dry with a soft towel.

If using as a body treatment, apply to your body while sitting in the tub, then rinse off in the shower. If need be, double the recipe, but you'll be surprised at how liquid the honey becomes when it is mixed with the fruit and warmed by your body.

Warm Wine Bath   (yang)

Chinese doctors have used wine on the body for ages. Because of its naturally acidic properties, wine is now being used by Western cosmetic companies. It has been re-named alpha-hydroxyl acid, and it comes with a hefty price tag! This warm wine bath will not only take away that chilled-to-the-bone feeling that comes with wintertime but also restore your skin's natural acid mantle. This is powerful protection against pollution and a great treatment for sunburn.

Makes 1 bath treatment

> 1 bottle white wine
> 1 cup coarse sea salt

Heat the wine in a saucepan while running the water into your tub. Dissolve the sea salt under the running water, and when the wine is hot, pour it into the tub.

Climb into the tub and soak. You'll be relaxed and warmed . . . especially if you've sampled some of the wine before adding it to your bath!

IF YOU HAVE OILY SKIN

Typically, those of you with oily skin have warmer (yang) tendencies. A higher level of oil secretion generally accompanies this. While women with this skin type are fortunate in that they often avoid fine lines and wrinkles, they do suffer from acne, skin problems such as blackheads and whiteheads, and enlarged pores. The goal of Chinese medicine is to cool down the internal organs and regulate oil production by eating the right foods and avoiding the wrong ones, and by using topical herbal treatments to cool the surface of the skin.

I recommend that clients who have oily skin consume the following fruits frequently: apples, bananas, dates, pears, plums, and strawberries. Fresh apple juice, with a slice of lemon if you like, can also be enjoyed, as well as pear, starfruit, strawberry, or watermelon juice. The following cool-energy vegetables are also excellent: carrots, cucumbers, daikon radishes, lettuce, peas, spinach, and water chestnuts. Herbs that help balance oily skin include chamomile, chrysanthemum, dandelion flowers, garlic, honeysuckle, and peppermint. Be sure to drink plenty of plain water to hydrate your body. Teas, juices, and soups help, but they're not the same.

If you have oily skin, avoid or eliminate the following foods: citrus fruits, sweet basil, cloves, Chinese parsley (coriander), caraway seeds, mangoes, and hot peppers. Avoid fried foods, fats, sweets, foods containing fungus and yeast, and processed foods, including most breads and pasta.

If your skin is oily, resist the temptation to use alcohol-based cleaning and toning products on your face. These will remove excess oil, to be sure, but will trick the sebaceous glands in your skin into thinking they have not done their job properly, because alcohol removes *too much* oil. As a result, these oil-producing glands will work overtime to make sure your skin—especially your face—has enough oil to stay pliant and moist. This sets off a vicious cycle that results in damaged, sometimes painful, skin. To keep this from happening, use cleansing products that soothe and cool the skin.

RECIPES FOR OILY SKIN

Cold Cucumber Soup *(yin)*

This is a splendid hot-weather soup with cooling properties that everyone will enjoy, regardless of skin type. It is especially good for those with oily skin and anyone who suffers from frequent rashes or skin irritation. You can jazz this up by adding a tomato, peeled and coarsely chopped.

Makes 4 appetizer or 2 main-dish servings

2 medium cucumbers
2 garlic cloves, peeled and chopped
1 small green bell pepper, seeded and coarsely chopped
1 small onion, peeled and quartered
A few small pieces of ice
1 teaspoon fresh lemon juice, or to taste
Salt and pepper, to taste

Peel cucumbers and cut them in half lengthwise. Using the tip of a spoon, scrape out the seeds and discard. Coarsely chop into 1-inch pieces. Place half of the cucumbers, garlic, bell pepper, onion, and a few pieces of ice in the container of a blender or food processor (the ice chills and helps liquefy the mixture). Process until the soup is somewhat smooth. Add the remaining half of the ingredients and process again. Season with lemon juice, salt, and pepper. Serve immediately in chilled soup bowls.

Barley–Strawberry Yogurt Scrub *(yin)*

The barley gently exfoliates without leaving your skin feeling raw like many commercial scrubs do. The yogurt maintains the skin's natural pH, which helps correct excess oil production. Strawberries are full of vitamin C, which applied topically, will help prevent skin from aging.

Makes 1 treatment

> ¼ cup raw barley flakes
> ½ cup strawberry yogurt

Process uncooked barley with the strawberry yogurt in a blender. Gently work into your skin, taking care to avoid the delicate tissues around the eyes. Leave on for 2 minutes, then rinse off with tepid water and pat face dry with a soft towel.

Chamomile-Mint Toner *(yin)*

Here is a wonderful, natural, alcohol-free toner you can safely apply to sensitive, broken-out areas several times a day. Chamomile and mint leaves are soothing to even the most sensitive skin. This light, fragrant liquid cools the hot energy that radiates from your skin and controls excess facial oil.

Makes 7 to 10 applications

> 1 tablespoon dried chamomile leaves (or 1 tea bag)
> 1 tablespoon dried mint or ¼ cup chopped fresh mint
> 1 tablespoon fresh lemon juice

Bring 2 cups of water to a rolling boil in a medium-sized glass or enamel saucepan, and add the chamomile and mint. Reduce heat to medium and simmer for 30 minutes, or until the liquid is reduced to ½ cup. Cool and strain liquid. Discard herbs. Add the lemon juice; stir to blend. Refrigerate in a glass bottle with a tightly fitting lid for up to one week.

To use, pour 1 to 2 tablespoons into a glass bowl and apply toner to the face with cotton balls once or twice a day (do not use directly from bottle to avoid contamination).

Honey-Lemon Moisturizing Treatment   (yin)

Although it may seem odd, honey has been used as a moisturizer for centuries. A natural humectant, it will heal abrasions, soothe roughness, and relieve redness without adding any unnecessary oils. Lemon is a natural astringent that complements the honey's action and restores the skin's natural acid mantle that soaps wash away. When used on damp skin, this moisturizer instantly liquefies and is not sticky.

Makes 1 treatment

> 1 tablespoon raw honey
> 1 tablespoon fresh lemon juice

Mix honey and lemon juice in a glass bowl. Wet your face, then gently massage the mixture into your skin. Leave on for 3 minutes. Rinse well with tepid water and pat face dry with a soft towel.

Chrysanthemum-Chamomile Mask   (yin)

For deep cleansing, use this softly scented chrysanthemum-chamomile mask to make sure that your skin is taut and toned. This is especially good for oily skin, as it cleans the pores without stimulating oil production. Use weekly for great results.

Makes 1 treatment

2 tablespoons dried chrysanthemum petals (see NOTE)
2 tablespoons dried chamomile flowers (see NOTE)
2 tablespoons dried dandelion flowers (see NOTE)
2 tablespoons dried mint
2 tablespoons buckwheat
2 tablespoons kaolin or French clay (see NOTE)

Grind the herbs and the buckwheat into a powder using either a mortar and pestle or a blender. Add the kaolin and 4 to 5 tablespoons of hot water, a tablespoon at a time, while mixing into a paste.

Apply as a facial mask once a week, taking care to avoid the delicate skin around the eyes. Let dry for 30 minutes. Rinse off with tepid water. Pat face dry with a soft towel.

NOTE: Kaolin and French clay are both available in health food stores and many large drugstores and cosmetics shops. The dried flowers are available at herb shops and many large health food stores or by mail order from the Resources listed on page 253.

IF YOU HAVE ACNE

Typically found in people with overactive oil glands, acne is the result of an excess secretion of oil on the surface of the skin that clogs pores and attracts germs to the skin's surface. This unhappy alliance prohibits proper production of the skin's natural oils and results in the bumps we call acne.

When acne appears it is usually the result of a high yang (hot-energy) syndrome, especially during adolescence. The recipes in this chapter can help tone down the fire-red blemishes of youth. Unfortunately, acne doesn't just plague the young. Consider Sandra, the attorney who came into my salon complaining of both acne *and* dry skin (page 81). Stress, hormonal imbalances, clogged pores, and radical climate changes can all cause acne, no matter what your age.

Although it is always tempting, you should never try to break those boil-like blemishes at home, as the unfortunate result may well be lifelong scarring. A dermatologist or licensed skin-care professional trained in extraction and sterilization is definitely worth the expense in this case. In addition to seeing a health-care professional, I also recommend taking a multivitamin complex. A vitamin program for acne should contain the following:

- Vitamin A, which reduces the amount of fatty substances or sebum in the skin that can block pores and cause blackheads
- Vitamin B complex, which calms the nerves
- Vitamin C, which dilates blood vessels and increases circulation

Ideally, these vitamins should come from natural sources—vitamin A from yellow fruits and vegetables, the B vitamins from meats and whole grains, and vitamin C from citrus fruits, rose hips, and other vegetables and fruits.

Naturally, you should consult a professional before starting any program of supplements. The minimum daily requirements of these vitamins, which you will find on the label, should be sufficient.

Even though they have cooling energy, bamboo shoots—which can be found in cans, sliced, or in chunks, in most Asian markets—are especially good skin detoxifiers. They have one drawback in that they have properties that cause bumps under the skin to erupt, so you won't want to eat them the day before a big date. When my sisters and I had the measles, our mother gave us bamboo shoots to bring out all the bumps at once rather than waiting for them to come out a few at a time. This speeded our recovery time. If you are acne-prone, I wouldn't recommend eating bamboo shoots but would, instead, work internally to cure the problem.

Many herbs also act as anti-acne agents. These include eucalyptus, garlic, honeysuckle blossoms, dandelion flowers, chickweed, goldenseal, calendula, marigold, myrrh, thyme, and yellow dock, to name a few. These herbs can be brewed as teas and consumed as one would any other tea.

Whatever your age, if you have acne breakouts, be sure to avoid spicy, fried foods and herbs like chives and star anise—which is easy to do in the standard American diet.

RECIPES FOR ACNE

Apple-Yogurt Smoothie (yin)

Pour this delicious drink into a tall glass and enjoy it once a day, especially when a skin flare-up occurs. It has a cool, calming energy to put out the fire that causes this problem. You can use any kind of plain yogurt—regular or nonfat—to ease your skin from the inside out.

Makes 1 serving

> 1 apple, peeled, cored, and coarsely chopped
> 1 cup plain yogurt
> 1 tablespoon honey

Process the apple with the yogurt and honey in a blender until smooth—you can add water to thin the smoothie, if desired.

Barley-Lime-Honey Cleanser (yin)

This gently abrasive, slightly acidic cleanser is ideal for the acne sufferer. It helps unclog pores and regulate the skin's oil production.

Makes 1 treatment

> 2 tablespoons raw barley flakes or oatmeal
> 2 tablespoons fresh lime juice
> 1 teaspoon raw honey

Mix the raw barley with the lime juice and let sit for 5 minutes while the barley softens; then add honey. Stir thoroughly. Apply to wet face and gently massage, taking care to avoid the delicate tissue around the eyes. Rinse with tepid water and pat face dry with a soft towel.

Sunset Citrus Splash   (yin)

This easy-to-make skin toner is especially good for anyone with acne or other skin problems usually associated with oily skin. It's astringent without being drying and adds vitamin C to tender blemishes to promote healing.

Makes 7 to 10 treatments

    1 vitamin C tablet, crushed
    1 lemon
    1 lime

Bring ½ cup of water to a boil. Remove from heat and add the crushed vitamin C tablet. Stir until dissolved. Allow to cool.

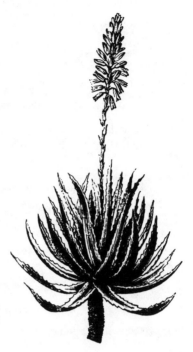

Aloe vera (*Aloe socotrina*)

    Squeeze the juice from the lemon and the lime and discard all seeds. Strain the juice into the cooled liquid, and stir until completely mixed. Pour into a small glass bottle, and store in the refrigerator until ready to use. To use, pour 1 to 2 tablespoons into a glass bowl and apply to the skin with cotton balls once or twice daily. Rinse with cool water before going out into the sun.

Lavender-Aloe Moisturizer   (yin)

Lavender is a natural antiseptic and antibacterial herb. Aloe vera juice soothes and promotes healing. Together, they help the skin hold moisture quite wonderfully.

Makes 1 treatment

2 tablespoons dried lavender (see NOTE)
1 tablespoon aloe vera juice

Bring ½ cup of water to a boil. Add the dried lavender and steep until cool. Strain and discard the flowers. Add the aloe to the liquid and stir thoroughly.

Apply with cotton balls to the face or the body as needed—it does not need to be rinsed off. It is particularly good if left on overnight. This moisturizer does not keep well—make a fresh batch each time.

NOTE: Dried lavender is available from most herb shops and health food stores or by mail order from the Resources listed on page 253.

Mint-Clay Mask   (yin)

This mask is perfect for reviving acne-plagued skin, especially after a night out. The mint cuts oil and stimulates skin, while the clay draws out oil and impurities from your skin.

Makes 1 treatment

1 teaspoon dried mint, or 1 mint tea bag
4 tablespoons kaolin or French clay (see NOTE)

Boil 1 cup of water and add the dried mint or tea bag. Steep until cool. Put the clay into a glass bowl, and add the peppermint tea, teaspoon by teaspoon, stirring until smooth—it should have the consistency of yogurt. Pat evenly on your face, avoiding the delicate tissue around the eyes, and on your body, as desired. Let dry 10 to 15 minutes. Rinse off, using tepid water, and pat skin dry with a soft towel.

NOTE: Kaolin and French clay are both available in health food stores and many large drugstores and cosmetics shops.

IF YOU HAVE DRY SKIN

Dry skin secretes less oil than other skin types. Women with this type of skin are more prone to fine lines and wrinkles. While dry skin is, in large part, hereditary, you can adjust this condition and improve the look of your parched epidermis almost immediately through diet.

Rachel is a great example of this problem. Thirty-five years old, five feet tall and a bit skinny, she was in my salon for a few moments before I even realized she was there. She was quite shy, and it took some intensive probing before she would answer my questions. Her younger sister was getting married within the week, and Rachel was feeling very old, as she saw every line on her face increase with each passing day. She wanted a quick cure, something that would miraculously restore what she felt was her rapidly fading youth.

Of course, I asked her first about her diet. She was so afraid of gaining weight, she had eliminated all fats and oils from her diet.

While most skin types are hereditary, there was much Rachel could do to help herself. The most difficult part was convincing her to add avocados and good oils to her diet. She promised to try them for a week, but that was all. I gave her a list of foods to eat and foods to avoid, and gave her some topical creams to help ease the pain of her dry skin. She was dubious when she left, but she had tried everything else. She decided that she might as well give this a try. By the end of the week, she called me with marvelous news. For the first time in years, she could wash her face without it hurting—her skin had been so dry that even the most gentle cleanser and water stung. She went to the wedding, feeling confident and looking radiant. She was so amazed by the results that she promised to stick to the program I had given her.

Your diet can have a marked effect in counterbalancing dry skin. The best foods to eat are adzuki beans, papaya, ginseng, dang quai, honey, black sesame seeds, sunflower seeds, black and yellow soybeans, and ginger. Also consider jelly-textured foods, which help to maintain the skin's elasticity—royal jelly, meat tendons, shark's fin, gelatin, and bone marrow are all natural elasticity boosters.

If you suffer from dry skin, you should eat less of the following foods, which can exacerbate the condition: apples, grapefruits, strawberries, pears, tomatoes, hops (a prime ingredient in beer), radishes, vinegar, and hard liquor.

RECIPES FOR DRY SKIN

Potato Soup (yin)

If your skin is especially dry and tender, you will benefit from a meal that starts with this amazing soup. Made with foods that are known to be balanced and cooling, this soup will ease painful itching and irritation.

Makes 6 appetizer or 4 main-dish servings

> 4 potatoes
> 1 onion
> 3 stalks celery
> 2 carrots
> 3 cloves garlic, peeled and chopped
> Salt and pepper to taste

Peel and chop the vegetables into ½-inch pieces. Place the vegetables and garlic in a large enamel saucepan and add 6 to 8 cups of water. Bring to a rolling boil. Reduce heat and simmer for 30 minutes to 1 hour, until the liquid is reduced by half. Season with salt and pepper.

Oatmeal-Honey Scrub (yin)

Oatmeal has long been used to soothe and nourish the skin while gently exfoliating it. You can cook it especially for this scrub, but I just put aside a little bit of my morning oatmeal and use that! The honey soothes, heals, and gives your skin much-needed moisture.

Makes 1 treatment

> 2 tablespoons raw honey
> 2 tablespoons cooked oatmeal

Mix the honey with the cooled oatmeal. Wet your face and gently massage the mixture into your face and neck, taking care to avoid the delicate tissue around the eyes. Rinse off with tepid water and pat face dry with a soft towel.

Slippery Elm Splash   (yin)

Slippery elm makes a great tea; use it when you've been speaking a lot or have a sore throat. It has also been used traditionally for lubricating without oil and for soothing abrasions. Rather than buying slippery elm bark and preparing it in a time-consuming process, I buy a widely marketed slippery elm tea at the health food store.

Makes 1 treatment

   1 teabag Throat-Coat tea (see NOTE)

Boil 1 cup of water and add tea bag. Steep until water is cool. Splash over face and body; this does not need to be washed off. However, this splash must be made fresh every time you use it.

NOTE: Throat-Coat tea is widely available in health food stores and in many drugstores and grocery stores.

Ginseng-Almond Luxury Lotion   (yin/yang)

Historically, ginseng has been more treasured than gold, for as the ancients said, it "holds the secret to eternal youth." Ginseng's health-fortifying qualities are legendary. Paired with the emollient properties of sweet almonds, this lotion will nourish and protect your dry skin from the elements.

Makes 8 to 10 applications

1 piece ginseng root, approximately 2 to 3 inches in length
½ cup almond oil
1 tablespoon honey
⅛ teaspoon baking soda
3 tablespoons grated beeswax
1 tablespoon liquid lanolin (see NOTE)
½ teaspoon almond extract

Pour 3 cups of water into a glass saucepan and add the whole ginseng root. Bring liquid to a boil, cover, reduce temperature, and simmer over low heat for 2 hours, or until root is soft and the liquid is reduced to 1 cup.

Remove root and set liquid aside. Chop the cooked ginseng root as finely as possible. Return chopped ginseng root and 1 cup ginseng liquid to saucepan and add the almond oil. Simmer gently about 1 hour, or until liquid is reduced to ½ cup. Let cool.

Strain the liquid into a glass bowl, discarding the ginseng. Add the honey, baking soda, grated beeswax, and liquid lanolin. Pour back into the saucepan and heat gently until the wax is melted. Stir to blend. When wax is thoroughly melted, add the almond extract and stir again.

Pour this mixture into a clean, dry glass jar. Allow to cool completely. Stir again, then cover. Store in refrigerator for 10 days to 2 weeks.

To use, massage lightly into the skin to restore moisture. Remove any excess with cotton balls. Use in the morning and again at night.

NOTE: Liquid lanolin is available in health food stores and many large drugstores.

Morning Star Detoxifying Mask   (yin)

Start your day off with this refreshing wake-up mask. I often used it on those mornings when I had long hours in front of the camera ahead of me. All dryness is erased, and my skin is left feeling and looking sparkling and soft . . . and free of aging toxins. If your skin is especially dry, you will find this alcohol-free toning mask especially helpful in removing wrinkles and easing dryness.

Makes 1 treatment

> 1 starfruit, coarsely chopped
> 1 teaspoon fresh lemon juice
> 3 to 4 tablespoons rice flour
> 3 tablespoons sweet almond oil

Place the starfruit in a glass bowl. Add the lemon juice and stir to mix. Add rice flour, a tablespoon at a time, and stir to mix. Add sweet almond oil to form an oatmeal-like paste.

Using your fingertips, pat this mixture onto your face, taking care to avoid the delicate tissue around your eyes. Leave on face for 10 minutes, then rinse off with tepid water, rubbing gently with a soft cloth. Pat face dry with a soft towel.

IF YOU HAVE COMBINATION SKIN

In the Chinese way of thinking, combination skin—when that T-shaped zone across your forehead and down your nose is oily and the rest of your face is dry or normal—may be a signal that your body is out of balance. Most skin-care products that are used to control oiliness are too harsh for the rest of your face, and products created for dry and normal skin are not effective when treating oiliness.

The good news is that once you have cleansed your body of toxins and begun to nourish and regenerate it so that it becomes balanced, this condition corrects itself. Whole foods and herbs have astounding properties that benefit the skin internally as well as topically.

Concentrate on foods that will act on the lungs and large intestines, the yin and yang organs relating to the skin, and the stomach and spleen, because of their roles in digestion and purification of the body. These predominantly yin and neutral foods include corn, spinach, lettuce, honey, beef, and celery.

RECIPES FOR COMBINATION SKIN

Honey-Mint-Barley Scrub   (yin)

This is a perfect, balanced scrub that will lubricate, moisturize, and soothe your skin. The honey adds needed moisture while not adding any oil, the peppermint is lightly astringent, tightening your skin, and the barley will gently slough off any dead skin cells.

Makes 1 treatment

> 1 tablespoon dried mint, or 1 tea bag
> 3 tablespoons honey
> 1 teaspoon barley

Boil 1 cup of water and add the dried mint or tea bag. Steep until cool. Strain and discard mint leaves or tea bag. Combine the honey and barley in a separate cup. Add the mint tea, a tablespoon at a time, until mixture forms a loose paste. Discard remaining tea.

Apply scrub to cleansed face and gently massage with your fingertips, taking care to avoid the delicate tissue around your eyes. Rinse face with tepid water and pat dry with a soft towel.

Parsley Toner   (yin)

Parsley is a good source of vitamin C, which has a gentle astringent property that helps equalize the pH balance of the skin. This soothing toner is perfect for combination skin and is particularly good for nighttime use.

Makes 2 treatments

> 1 large bunch parsley, coarsely chopped

Bring ½ cup of water to a boil. Place parsley in a large glass bowl, and add the boiling water; let steep until cool. Strain the liquid and store in a glass bottle with a tight-fitting lid in the refrigerator.

Apply cool toner to face with cotton balls; this can be left on skin without rinsing. Discard mixture after 2 days.

Raw-Honey Moisturizing Treatment   (yin/yang)

The most important ingredient you can have in your "skin food" cupboard is raw honey. The propolis in honey is a free-radical neutralizer and is full of vitamins C, B, and E. It is extremely important to use raw honey, which can be found in any health food store, because these nutrients are not present in the pasteurized honey on the supermarket shelves. If you have only pasteurized honey, try it, but raw honey is far more effective. Honey adds no oil to your skin, but instead tricks your skin into minimizing the overproduction of oils. Honey soothes and lubricates both the oily and the dry parts of your combination skin.

Makes 1 treatment

    2 tablespoons raw honey

Place 2 tablespoons raw honey in a cup and stir in 1 to 2 teaspoons of water. Pat onto your damp skin, gently massaging it into your face and neck with your fingertips. Leave on for 3 minutes, then rinse off with tepid water. Pat face dry with a soft towel.

Bay Leaf and Clay Mask   (yin/yang)

Bay leaves have been used to normalize skin for hundreds of years. They have both stimulating and soothing component oils and are a natural antibacterial agent. The clay will draw out any impurities that are in your skin, leaving it clean, fresh, and smooth.

Makes 1 treatment

3 or 4 dried bay leaves

3 or 4 tablespoons kaolin or French clay (see NOTE)

Bring 1 cup of water to a boil. Put the bay leaves into a glass bowl and add the boiling water; let stand until cool. Put the clay into a small bowl and spoon the bay leaf water, tablespoon by tablespoon, into the clay until it is the consistency of a milkshake. Pat evenly onto your face and/or body with your fingertips. Let dry for about 20 minutes, then rinse off with tepid water. Pat skin dry with a soft towel.

NOTE: Kaolin and French clay are both available in health food stores and many large drugstores and cosmetics shops.

IF YOU HAVE SENSITIVE OR ALLERGIC SKIN

Sensitive or allergic skin indicates an imbalance in the large intestine, which play a major role in the water balance of the body and the purity of the body's fluids. The large intestine—the yang organ opposite the yin organ of the lungs—has special influence over the throat, face, and head. The large intestine helps rid the body of toxins likely to cause skin sensitivity or allergic reactions.

The simplest, most direct way to eliminate toxins is to perspire, so you can either steam toxins from your face—a recipe for Honeysuckle Skin Steam follows on page 110—or eat foods that encourage perspiration, such as dishes that include ginger or pepper. Possibly the most helpful ingredients in any treatment for sensitive skin are honey, honeysuckle, and chrysanthemum flowers.

Louisa, a very pale blonde, often broke out in "little itchy bumps" on her upper arms, chest, and face. She asked what to do to clear up these irritating bumps and to heal the ones she had scratched during her sleep. It was summertime and far too hot to wear long sleeves, but the sores on her arms were both painful and unsightly. Exposure to sun and airborne pollutants only exacerbated the condition. I suggested that she rub raw honey onto the irritated areas, explaining that honey is soothing and healing. A humectant that lubricates and moisturizes the skin, honey also has antibacterial and antibiotic properties.

RECIPES FOR SENSITIVE OR ALLERGIC SKIN

Vinegar Tea   (yang)

This tasty drink may sound a bit peculiar to Westerners, but I'm sure you will appreciate what it does to calm and cool hot, burning skin from the inside out by opening the pores and encouraging perspiration. This tea is especially helpful for anyone who breaks out in a rash after eating seafood.

Makes 1 serving

> 1-inch piece ginger, peeled and halved
> ¼ cup red wine vinegar
> 1 tablespoon brown sugar

Combine ¼ cup of water with the remaining ingredients in a small glass or enamel saucepan. Bring to a boil, then lower the flame and simmer for 10 minutes. Strain, and drink the tea while still warm.

Green Mung Bean Seaweed Soup   (yin)

Green mung beans have the exact opposite energy of red beans. This wonderful soup clears the excess hot energy that causes imbalance. It also works as a diuretic and has been shown to lower blood pressure. It is especially helpful for problems relating to sensitive skin.

Makes 6 appetizer or 4 main-dish servings

1 strip dried seaweed—kombu, arame, or kelp (see NOTE)
½ pound dried green mung beans, washed and trimmed
   of tough ends
1 teaspoon sugar

Soak the seaweed strip in hot water for 5 minutes; then wash and cut it into strips.

Bring 4 cups of water to a boil in a medium-sized enamel saucepan. Add green mung beans and seaweed, lower the heat, and simmer for ½ hour, or until the beans are tender. Add the sugar.

NOTE: Dried seaweed and green mung beans are available from Asian markets and health food stores.

Egg White and Honey Cleanser   (yin/yang)

Honey is particularly good for sensitive skin, as it soothes, moisturizes, and cleans the skin without causing any irritation. The addition of an ancient beauty ingredient—egg whites—further calms your sensitive epidermis.

Makes 1 treatment

   2 tablespoons raw honey
   1 tablespoon whipped egg whites

Mix the honey and egg whites together in a cup, then gently massage into your skin, using your fingertips to avoid stretching the skin. Leave on for 3 minutes, so that the honey can draw out the impurities. Rinse your face with tepid water and pat dry with a soft towel.

Comfrey-Raspberry Splash   (yin)

The old-fashioned name for comfrey is "knit-bone," which bespeaks its role in cell regeneration. Raspberry is a gentle astringent full of needed vitamin C that is so healing to sensitive and allergic skin.

Makes 2 applications

    1 tablespoon dried comfrey, or 1 tea bag (see NOTE)
    1 tablespoon dried raspberry tea or 1 tea bag (see NOTE)

Bring 1 cup of water to a boil and pour over the dried comfrey and raspberry tea in a glass bowl. Let steep until cool. Remove tea bag or strain leaves. Pour into a glass bottle with a tightly fitting lid and refrigerate until ready to use. Pour half the liquid into a glass bowl. Using cotton balls, gently pat your skin with the liquid; it does not need to be rinsed off.

NOTE: Dried comfrey and dried raspberry leaves are available at health food stores and herb shops or by mail order from the Resources listed on page 253.

Honey-Avocado Body Moisturizer   (yin/yang)

Avocados provide an easily assimilated oil that mimics the body's own natural oils, yet does not clog the pores. The skin is your largest organ, and it's important to re-member that any pesticide that is sprayed on the avocado will be absorbed immediately into your epidermis. So, it is really important that you get an organic avocado and raw honey. This moisturizing treatment is so soothing to sensitive skin, it'll make you feel like you've been to a spa!

Makes 1 total body treatment

    1 ripe avocado, peeled and pitted
    ½ cup raw honey

Process avocado and honey into a thick paste in a blender. Pour into a plastic bowl or cup (no glass, lest you drop it into the tub or shower). Take a warm shower; rinsing thoroughly to make sure there are no pollutants or soap on your body. Rub some of the avocado-honey paste all over your body and relax for 5 minutes. Rinse off the paste with tepid water. Pat your body dry with a soft towel.

Clay-Milk Mask   (yin/yang)

As a perfect weekly treatment for sensitive, allergic skin, this mask is a boon. The clay draws out impurities, while the milk soothes tender skin. It's so gentle you can use it more often if your skin is especially irritated.

Makes 1 treatment

> 3 tablespoons kaolin or French clay (see NOTE)
> 2 to 3 tablespoons milk or cream

Place clay in a glass cup or bowl. Stir in milk or cream until the mixture has a smooth, runny consistency. Pat onto clean skin, avoiding the delicate tissue around the eyes. Let dry for 15 to 20 minutes. Rinse face off with cool (not cold) water and pat dry with a soft towel.

NOTE: Kaolin or French clay is available in most health food stores and in many large drugstores and cosmetics shops.

Honeysuckle Skin Steam   (yin)

Honeysuckle blossoms are used in many Chinese facial creams for their superior ability to clear up acne and other skin irritations. Regardless of your skin type—oily, dry, normal, or acne prone—a fragrant steam of these delicate dried flowers will soothe your tender epidermis and facilitate your skin's ability to achieve a healthy balance.

Makes 1 facial steam

¼ cup dried honeysuckle blossoms, or 4 honeysuckle
    tea bags (see NOTE)

Bring 2 cups of water to a boil. Put the honeysuckle blossoms or tea bags in
a glass bowl and slowly pour the boiling water over them. Cover the bowl
with a small towel and let steep for 2 minutes.

To steam your face: Place bowl on a solid surface. Lift the towel and
place it over your head. Lean over the bowl and let the warm vapors hydrate
your skin for up to 10 minutes, or until liquid cools. Discard liquid.

Pat face dry with a soft towel. Follow up with a good moisturizer if you
have dry or normal skin. Use a toner or splash if your skin is oily or acne
prone.

NOTE: Dried honeysuckle is available at herb shops and health food stores,
or by mail order from the Resources listed on page 253.

IF YOU HAVE ECZEMA

Although eczema is a very common skin problem, its precise causes and a uni-
versally effective treatment continue to elude Western medical practitioners.
Chinese herbal practitioners believe eczema results from wind conditions and
exposure to extreme temperatures, and they treat it accordingly.

Eczema can appear on the face, behind the ears, on the upper arms, or on
other parts of the body. Wherever eczema occurs, unattractive reddish sores appear that can be painful, itchy, or sore. These patches can vanish mysteriously,
then reappear, all within a few days. Left untreated, eczema can result in thick,
rough spots that are as uncomfortable as they are unsightly.

Marlene came into my spa in search of something to treat the unsightly red
patches that had erupted behind her ears and on the backs of her hands. The
blotches, which had begun to spread, were painful and itchy. She was reluctant to
try the cortisone and steroid treatment her dermatologist had recommended.
"Those are powerful drugs," she said. "It seems like overkill to me."

As we talked, Marlene mentioned that she had just started her own business and was working around the clock to make a go of it. Picking up on that, I asked when she started her company and when the eczema started. Marlene opened her eyes wide and said, "I never thought about it, but I started breaking out right after I left my old job."

I explained to Marlene that eczema is an indication that the body has a yang *chi* excess that is often intensified by stress and anxiety. We discussed relaxation techniques for her to try and ways that she could alter her diet to restore balance to her body. I also suggested some natural remedies to relieve the itching and cool the hot energy in her body.

The following foods and herbs calm the wind conditions associated with eczema: peas, witch hazel, honey, ginger, chamomile, and thyme. Incorporate them into your diet and skin-care routines. For example, stir-fry snow peas with tofu and ginger, add green peas to soups or salads, and drink chamomile tea or use it as a toner. Incorporate these foods and you'll quickly see results. Drink plenty of water.

Conversely, the following foods should be assiduously avoided by those suffering from eczema: milk and all dairy products, yeast, sugar, mangoes, pineapples, strawberries, mustard greens, and shellfish. Chicken should be eaten only in moderation.

RECIPES FOR ECZEMA

Bee Pollen and Honey Pick-Me-Up   (yin/yang)

The synergy between bee pollen and honey make this a powerful morning tonic for anyone suffering from eczema or any other chronic skin problem. Honey is a humectant that lubricates the digestive tract and opens the flow of chi throughout the body. Drink every morning during episodes of eczema.

Makes 1 serving

    2 tablespoons honey
    2 tablespoons bee pollen (see NOTE)
    1 tablespoon ginseng extract (see NOTE)

Heat 1 cup of water to medium-hot but not boiling and pour into a large mug. Add honey, bee pollen, and ginseng extract. Stir well, and drink.

NOTE: Bee pollen and ginseng extract are both available at health food stores.

Papaya Peanut Soup   (yin/yang)

This tasty soup not only helps dry skin but also combats rashes, eczema, and other skin irritations as well. It's also good for strengthening the stomach and spleen, thus clearing heat and aiding the elimination process. Enjoy this soup often and experience beautiful, soft skin and better digestion.

Makes 2 main-dish servings

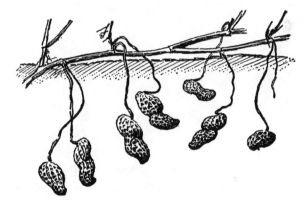

Peanuts (*Arachis hypogaea*)

> ½ pound lean pork, cut into ½-inch cubes
> 1 ripe papaya, peeled, seeded, and cut into 1-inch pieces
> 4 ounces unsalted raw peanuts, rinsed and skins removed
> Salt to taste

Season the pork with a pinch of salt. Put all ingredients into a pot, bring to a boil, and lower the heat to medium for about 20 minutes. Add salt to taste.

Papaya-Yogurt Body Scrub   (yin)

You shouldn't eat papaya and yogurt if you have eczema, but that shouldn't stop you from using this fragrant and refreshing body scrub to bring your skin into balance. Not only is papaya one of the best cooling summer fruits, being very yin, it also works miracles on dull, flaky skin and helps combat eczema. Enzymes in the papaya invigorate the skin, and the yogurt's natural acids work to gently remove old, dead skin cells so that new, healthy ones can emerge.

Makes 1 facial or skin treatment

    ½ cup chopped papaya
    ½ cup plain yogurt

Combine papaya and yogurt in a glass bowl and mix thoroughly. Apply to face, elbows, knees, feet—anywhere your skin needs softening or where eczema appears—and leave on for 10 minutes. Rinse skin with tepid water and pat dry with a soft towel.

Thyme-Lavender Toner   (yin/yang)

Thyme is an excellent emollient, and at the same time works to slough off dead skin cells and bring healing energy to patches of eczema. Lavender is particularly great for its soothing and antibiotic actions.

Makes 4 treatments

    1 tablespoon dried thyme
    1 tablespoon dried lavender (see NOTE)

Bring 1 cup of water to a boil. Place thyme and lavender in a large mug, and cover with water. Steep until cold. Strain off liquid and discard leaves. Pour the liquid into a glass bottle with a tightly fitting top. Store in the refrigerator for up to a week.

To use, pour ¼ cup into a bowl. Apply to face and body with cotton balls after bathing. This does not have to be washed off; in fact, it's particularly good as a pre-makeup toner.

NOTE: Dried lavender is available at herb shops and health food stores.

Chamomile-Aloe Moisturizer   (yin)

Aloe vera is one of the oldest recorded healing herbs, and chamomile has great soothing properties, making this an important moisturizer for eczema-plagued skin. It can be left on overnight or used under makeup for all-day protection.

Makes 1 treatment

> 1 tablespoon dried chamomile, or 1 tea bag
> 3 tablespoons aloe vera gel

Bring ½ cup of water to a boil. Pour water over the dried chamomile or tea bag in a glass bowl or cup. Steep until water is cool, then strain off liquid and discard the chamomile.

In a separate cup, add the aloe vera gel to 3 tablespoons of the chamomile tea. Mix well. Discard remaining tea. Apply to face and/or body with cotton balls.

Comfrey, Honey, and Egg Mask   (yin/yang)

This mask is great for the special needs of eczema sufferers. The comfrey aids cellular regeneration, the honey adds antibiotic and moisturizing properties, and the egg tightens the skin very gently. Use on your face and on any areas where eczema appears.

Makes 1 treatment

1 tablespoon dried comfrey, or 1 tea bag (see NOTE)
2 tablespoons raw honey
1 whole egg

Bring 1 cup of water to a boil. Pour the boiling water over the dried comfrey or tea bag in a glass bowl. Let steep until cool; strain and discard comfrey.

In a separate glass cup, mix the honey, egg, and ¼ cup of the cooled
comfrey tea. Discard remaining tea. Pat the mixture on clean face; leave on
for 5 minutes, or until skin feels taut. Rinse face with warm water, and pat
dry with a soft towel.

NOTE: Dried comfrey is available at herb shops and health food stores.

IF YOU HAVE LIVER SPOTS

Usually beginning in middle age, liver spots can appear on the face or the hands.
Typically darker than the skin's own shade, they range in color from light to dark
brown and from light to dark gray. Chinese herbalists believe that liver spots are
the result of liver imbalances.

My mother returned to live in Hong Kong after some twenty years in the
United States. Whenever I visit her there, I love going out with her on her morning walks. A neighbor, Mrs. Stone, is the wife of an American businessman now
working in Hong Kong. For a few years, she and my mother have met for their
early-morning walks along the trails in the hills where they live. Even though my
mother is about ten years older than Mrs. Stone, my mother is more fit—and her
hands are softer and more beautiful than her friend's.

One morning, during my last visit, Mrs. Stone told me that she had noticed
my mother's beautiful hands and had asked Mom how she did it. My mother's
friend had quite a few dark-brown liver spots on her hands, which made her self-
conscious. The skin was dry, like paper, with pronounced veins.

Always willing to share her knowledge about traditional Chinese medicine
and herbal beauty treatments, Mom gave her a few tips. She showed her how to

care for her hands and nails and told her how to make minor changes in her diet to nurture and cleanse her liver and kidneys that would be especially effective in removing those ugly spots. Mom also told Mrs. Stone to follow her lead and wear thin white cotton gloves when she goes on her morning walks. Now they both apply a lot of moisturizer and pull on their cotton gloves before their walks.

When I last saw her, Mrs. Stone proudly showed off the results of her efforts. Her hands looked about ten years younger, and you could hardly see the liver spots at all. When I made a comment about how pretty her hands were, she was very happy and proud to acknowledge my mother's wise advice.

RECIPES THAT LIGHTEN LIVER SPOTS

Papaya Bleaching Scrub   (yin/yang)

Papaya's natural enzymes soften the skin while exfoliating and bleaching it. Lemon is a great source of much-needed vitamin C and is also a great bleach. Honey moisturizes and revitalizes.

Makes 1 treatment

> 1 ripe papaya
> 1 lemon, juiced
> 1 tablespoon raw honey

Peel the papaya and place in a bowl. Mash thoroughly, then add the lemon juice and honey. Mix well, and rub on skin. Leave on for 5 minutes, rinse off, and pat skin dry with a soft towel.

Eucalyptus–Witch Hazel–Lemon Toner   (yin)

The eucalyptus lends this toner wonderful antiseptic qualities, and the witch hazel and lemon both act as bleaching agents. Used regularly, this toner will help lighten liver spots.

Makes 4 treatments

> 5 drops eucalyptus oil
> 1 lemon, juiced
> 8-ounce bottle witch hazel

Add the eucalyptus oil and the lemon juice to the bottle of witch hazel. Shake well.

Pour ¼ cup of the solution into a glass bowl. Using cotton balls, apply to the affected areas. Store the toner in refrigerator for up to 7 days.

Happy Honeysuckle Oil   (yin)

This is particularly good for softening the tough, old-looking skin that frequently accompanies liver spots. Honeysuckle not only smells wonderful, it also has hydrating properties that keep skin dewy. Rub a little of this sensational oil onto your legs after shaving! You'll be amazed at how soft your skin will stay.

Makes 4 ounces

> 3 tablespoons dried honeysuckle
>   flowers (see NOTE)
> 2 tablespoons liquid lecithin (see NOTE)
> ¼ cup olive oil
> 1 tablespoon wheat germ oil (see NOTE)
> 1 teaspoon oil of honeysuckle
>   (see NOTE)

Bring ¼ cup water to a boil and pour into a bowl. Add the honeysuckle flowers and steep until cool. Set aside.

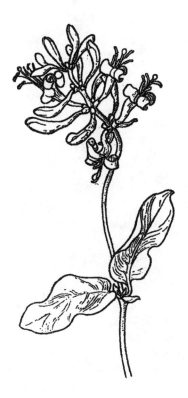

Honeysuckle (*Lonicera hispidula*)

Process lecithin and oils in a blender at medium speed for 1 minute. Strain and discard the honeysuckle flowers from the liquid, then add the liquid to the oil mixture in the blender. Process for 1 minute at low speed.

Pour into a clean, dry glass container. Store tightly sealed in a cool, dark place. Shake before use, as it may separate. Rub oil into skin wherever necessary.

NOTE: All ingredients noted can be found in health food stores.

Supersweet Spot-Removing Mask   (yin/yang)

This lovely liquid emollient is excellent for liver spots. The sugar gently scrubs away dead skin cells, the lemon juice bleaches the spots, and the honey is a natural rehydrator for all skin types. Use weekly to help reduce the color of the spots.

Makes 1 treatment

> 1 tablespoon raw honey
> 3 tablespoons brown sugar
> 1 tablespoon fresh lemon juice

Mix together the honey, brown sugar, and lemon juice in a small cup. Wet the area to be scrubbed; then rub in the mixture. Let it stay on your skin for a few minutes to allow the bleaching and hydrating actions to occur; then rinse off with warm water and pat skin dry with a soft towel.

PROTECT YOUR SKIN FROM THE SUN

The only way to truly protect your skin from the sun is to stay indoors.

Of course, that's not practical. In ancient China, women always carried parasols to protect their skin from the "vicious elements," since a fair complexion was highly prized. Today, even as more and more evidence appears about the extensive damage the sun can do, a tan is still considered beautiful.

Why people knowingly put themselves and their skin in jeopardy is a puzzle to me. Even as women educate themselves about the dangers of unprotected sun exposure, cases of skin cancer increase, and the number of young adults consulting plastic surgeons for chemical peels and surgical procedures to remove wrinkles and restore youth to their faces is on the rise.

Since there is no surefire way for most of us to have a full, rich life without exposing ourselves to the sun, I make these suggestions:

- Always use a sunscreen with an SPF (sun protection factor) of at least fifteen. If you perspire heavily or will be in and out of the water, reapply it frequently during the day.
- Always wear a hat with a bill or brim to further protect your hair, scalp, and face from the sun.
- Use skin-care and cosmetic products that contain a sunscreen. The SPF will be printed on the label.
- To have a golden, sun-kissed tan, use a self-tanning product. There are several new products on the market that, used properly, look quite natural. You might also try a bronzing powder.

If you do get a burn or if you are already tanned and have the first signs of premature aging, you can stop what you're doing . . . and begin to take special care of this most visible part of your body. The recipes that follow provide a good place to start.

RECIPES FOR SUN-DAMAGED SKIN

Oatmeal Water–Vinegar Wash   (yin)

Oatmeal is great for softening and soothing sun-damaged skin. You can use a bit of your leftover breakfast oatmeal or you can use instant oatmeal to make this soothing cleansing product. The vinegar restores the skin's delicate acid mantle and eases tenderness.

Makes 1 treatment

3 tablespoons cooked oatmeal

1 teaspoon apple cider vinegar

Bring 1 cup of water to a boil. Add the cooked oatmeal to the water and stir to combine. The oatmeal will sink to the bottom of the cup, but just keep stirring it for about 3 minutes to make a watery paste. The oatmeal essence will permeate the water. Let the water cool, then strain, and discard any oatmeal. Add the vinegar. Apply to sunburned skin with cotton balls; do not rinse off.

Lettuce-Water Splash   (yin)

Lettuce water is an old recipe for sunburned skin. In addition to being soothing, the cooked lettuce has chemicals that help ease sunburn pain.

Makes 1 treatment

½ head of organic lettuce, any variety

Chop the lettuce coarsely, and place in a saucepan. Cover with 1 cup of water. Bring to a boil, then turn off the heat. Let the mixture stand until cool; strain. Apply to sunburned areas with cotton balls and do not rinse off. Since this splash does not keep; make a new batch each time you want to treat your skin.

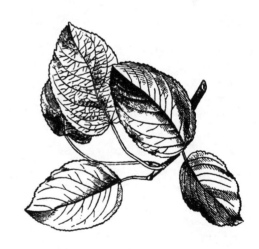

Tea leaves (*Pyrus communis*)

Aloe–Green Tea Moisturizer   (yin)

One of the most crucial methods to prevent sun damage—apart from sunscreen—is to restore moisture to seared skin cells. The tannic acid in the tea and the healing properties of the aloe vera gel make this simple brew an important tool in your sun-damage repair kit.

Makes 1 treatment

1 tablespoon loose green tea leaves, or 1 tea bag
2 tablespoons aloe vera gel

Bring 1 cup of water to a boil and pour over the green tea in a glass or crockery bowl. Steep until cool. Strain and discard tea. Add the aloe vera gel, mixing thoroughly. Apply to affected areas with cotton balls. Since this mixture does not keep, make a new batch each time.

Honey-Aloe Mask   (yin)

If your skin is sunburned, you definitely don't want to use any heavily astringent mask, as it will only cause more damage. This gentle mask will draw out impurities while utilizing the moisturizing qualities of honey.

Makes 1 treatment

2 tablespoons honey
2 tablespoons aloe vera gel

Stir honey and aloe vera gel together in a glass cup. Apply to affected areas. Leave on for 5 minutes, then rinse off with tepid water. Pat skin dry with a soft towel. This does not keep well, so make a new batch each time.

Dang Quai Damage Control Cream   (yang)

You have probably heard of dang quai as an herb that helps PMS and cramps. What you may not know is that it has superior healing properties, especially in the case of skin injuries. The Chinese use it in creams to help prevent the formation of thick, ugly scars. Here's a recipe that will soften dry skin and, thanks to its natural antibiotic qualities, promote healing and east the pain of sunburn.

Makes 6 to 8 treatments

1 slice dang quai, approximately 3 × 5 inches (see NOTE)
1 cup cocoa butter

Put enough water in a saucepan to touch the bottom of a steamer when placed on top of pan. Place the dang quai into the steamer. Cover the steamer and bring water to a boil. Reduce heat and simmer until dang quai is limp, approximately 10 minutes, depending on thickness of the root.

Remove the dang quai from steamer and discard water or sweeten with honey and drink. When dang quai is cool, chop the steamed root as finely as possible and set aside.

Place the cocoa butter and chopped dang quai in a saucepan and, over low heat, cook until the cocoa butter is thoroughly melted. Remove from heat. Cover loosely and let stand overnight.

The next day, heat again over low heat until the cocoa butter is melted. Strain through a metal sieve into a glass bowl. You may have to strain several times to remove all the pieces of dang quai.

Pour into a clean, dry glass container with a tightly fitting lid (allow to cool completely before sealing). Store in a cool, dark place for up to 10 days. Smooth the cream onto all affected areas.

NOTE: Dang quai is available at Asian markets and health food stores or by mail order from the Resources listed on page 253.

Mandarin Miracle Body Cream   (yin/yang)

Here's a natural cream that's good for any skin type. Mandarin Miracle Body Cream has a safflower oil base, which is neither too yin nor too yang, so it can be used all over your body. The orange peel helps to lighten any discolorations. This cream is especially good for softening those rough spots on your elbows, knees, and heels, and works very well to rehydrate sunburned skin.

Makes 4 to 6 treatments

2 teaspoons grated fresh orange peel
¼ cup safflower oil
1 tablespoon grated beeswax
¼ cup orange flower water (see NOTE)
Pinch of borax
1 teaspoon essential oil of orange (see NOTE)

Set aside 1 teaspoon of the grated orange peel. Combine safflower oil, remaining teaspoon of grated orange peel, and beeswax in a enamel or glass saucepan. Cook over low heat until beeswax is melted.

Combine the orange flower water with the borax in a second saucepan. Heat until water is warm and borax is completely dissolved. Pour this liquid into the beeswax and safflower oil mixture, add the teaspoon of grated orange peel and the oil of orange, and stir to combine.

Pour into a clean, dry glass container with a lid, allowing the mixture to cool completely before sealing. Store in a cool, dry place and use within 4 weeks. Smooth cream on all affected areas.

NOTE: Orange flower water and oil of orange are available at herb shops and health food stores.

6.

RECIPES FOR HEALTHY HAIR

YOU NEED MUCH MORE THAN A GREAT CUT

When I was a child—before my family came to the United States—I thought everybody had hair like mine. Certainly everyone I knew—my family, my neighbors, my schoolmates—had straight, relatively thick, black hair. Imagine my surprise when I saw the myriad colors, textures, and types of hair in the United States.

As I grew up, and especially after I began modeling, hair became a major concern: how it was styled, how it was cut, but most importantly the condition it was in.

In any culture, thick, healthy, radiant hair is a mark of beauty for which we all strive. Is it any wonder, then, that shampoos and conditioners are the biggest single category of beauty products marketed around the world?

Today, women and men alike spend massive amounts of time and money on their hair. And with good reason: hair frames the face. It is one of the first things people notice—the blue-eyed blonde; the little redhead; the tall, dark, handsome stranger.

Hair, like skin, is one of the first places our bodies manifest stress and illness. Shiny hair stands as a symbol of good health and serves as a "fashion accessory" even when we don't have on a stitch of makeup—or clothing. Still, in the West, use of hair as a diagnostic tool, as a reflection of the body's state of wellness, is relatively uncommon. In China, we scrutinize the hair and scalp for clues to our state of health.

WHAT WE DO TO OUR HAIR

We perm our hair, bleach it, straighten it, streak it, braid it, pull it, and spray it. We twist it around curling irons and heated rollers or blast it with dryers. Unless we take special precautions to fend off any damage with the many products manufactured to restore the moisture and oils, we are left with brittle, dry, dull, weak hair, and for more and more women, excessive hair loss.

Sarah, who is in her fifties, has fine, straight, naturally blond hair with silvery highlights. It is such a stunning color that she has been stopped on the street and asked who colors her hair. She was diagnosed as diabetic in her late forties, but she is generally in good health. Earlier this year, she noticed that her hair, which was usually shiny and bouncy, had become dull and limp. In fact, it was looking gray and drab rather than shining gold and silver, and she didn't like it one bit. At first, she wrote this off as a sign of aging and decided to discuss coloring her hair the next time she had it cut.

Sarah's stylist did not immediately jump at the prospect of coloring Sarah's hair. He noticed that since her last cut six weeks earlier, it had become dry, almost brittle, and appeared to be considerably thinner on top than it had been on her last visit. He could tell by touch that the cuticle, or outer layer, of Sarah's hair was rough. The cuticle, which is composed of transparent cells that look like overlapping shingles, was damaged, as was the second layer—the cortex—which contains the pigments that give hair its natural color. The dry, brittle feel also told him that the medulla, or middle layer, which determines the strength, body, and elasticity of the hair, was in a weakened condition. Apparently something was happening to deplete Sarah's vibrant color, turn her hair gray, and thin it out.

This savvy stylist asked Sarah what had been going on in her life: Had she been ill? Was she under a lot of stress at work or at home? What had she been eating lately? A lot of red meats and fried foods, shellfish, salt?

When Sarah told me her story, she said, "I was shocked. How did he know that from looking at my hair? I had been fighting a urinary tract infection for two or three weeks and was working around the clock to save an important account. I'd flown to Los Angeles and back and to London and back twice in the past month, and my meals had been sporadic to say the least. In L.A. I ate shrimp and crab legs, and in London, prime rib with all the trimmings. At home, I was living on danish and coffee, or cheese and crackers."

I explained to Sarah that according to Chinese theory, hair loss and premature graying were signs that the kidneys were not functioning properly, generally because of excessive hot energy. Inordinate stress, such as Sarah was experiencing with her quick trips to Los Angeles and London, can also result in stagnation of the spleen *chi,* another reason for loss of hair color. This hot-energy condition could be corrected by adding the cooling energy of *yin* foods to her diet.

Within two weeks of changing her diet to include more foods with cooling energy that nurture her kidneys, and eliminating those that interrupt the flow of *chi,* Sarah reported that her hair was already returning to health. Within a month, its golden silver color was back.

THE CHINESE APPROACH TO HAIR CARE

The road to stunning hair does not begin from without; it begins with our internal health. To the Chinese, hair that is anything other than shiny, strong, and healthy is not normal. Usually, it is an indication that the lungs and large intestines—the organs related to the skin and hair—are out of balance (see the chart on page 29).

Hair loss or weak, lifeless hair, accompanied by dry skin, insomnia, irritability, and nervousness, indicates deficient internal *yin* energy. By restoring this cooling energy to your system, you will quell the intense internal *yang* heat and bring balance to your body.

The large intestine, the *yang* organ associated with the hair, and the lungs, the *yin* organ that helps distribute moisture throughout the body, control the purity of the fluids in the body. As you know from the chart on page 29, the lungs are associated with the element metal, which nurtures water. The *yin* organ associated with water is the kidneys, so the lungs nurture the kidneys. Chinese practitioners study the hair and scalp to determine the condition of the blood and blood-cleansing organs, especially the kidneys. When there is an excess of protein, acids, fat, or toxins in the bloodstream, the hair follicles or roots do not receive enough nutrients to support growth. Severe hair loss—alopecia—often results, as does premature graying. As women age, a decline in estrogen levels also retards new hair growth.

To correct these problems, begin by rehydrating the blood and body fluids so that blood circulation to the scalp is increased. This is the only way nutrients can reach the hair follicle for continued new hair growth. Tonics and foods that nourish the blood, bone marrow, liver, and kidneys help make this happen. A list of these foods appears later in this chapter.

Healthy, shiny hair is a direct function of good circulation and healthy kidneys. Anything else—dandruff; dry, brittle hair; oily hair and scalp; weakened hair; balding or excessive hair loss—is a consequence of imbalance. Poor blood and *chi* results in a negative essence that causes hair to appear like a dying plant: dry, hard, and gloss-free. Adding the foods and herbs I'll discuss will help promote good circulation, strengthen the blood, and balance *chi,* all of which have beautiful and noticeable effects on the shine and strength of the hair.

THE NATURAL CYCLE OF HAIR GROWTH

Throughout our lives, our hair grows in cycles determined by nature and by our own body rhythms. Underneath every hair on your head is a new hair follicle beginning to grow. As it matures, this new hair shaft pushes the preceding hair out of the scalp. It is quite normal to lose between eighty and one hundred hairs a day—so few you hardly notice it—throughout most of our lives. More than this indicates that your body is out of balance.

Generally, we all are blessed as children with wonderful hair. If, however, we suffer before our mid-thirties from hair loss, premature graying, brittle or dry hair, or an extremely oily or dry scalp, we probably have poor kidney function. Liver function is also critical, and poor circulation subverts the state of our *chi,* which, in turn, wreaks havoc on our hair. As we age, a decline in estrogen levels retards the growth of new hair. In addition, an increase in sebaceous oils causes our hair to thin and gray—too much oil clogs the pores and kills hair follicles, causing hair to die and fall out. In women, this often begins with menopause.

Healthy sebaceous glands in the scalp are essential for healthy hair, since the oil these tiny glands produce lubricates the hair and scalp. Oily hair results from these glands secreting too much oil; dry hair, from too little. Brushing your hair helps stimulate the sebaceous glands and is recommended for men and women with dry hair. Those with oily hair should brush less. It should also come as no surprise that blow-drying and other hot-styling techniques are major contributors to dry, damaged, hair. I promise that if you set your dryer on the cool setting, you will see a major improvement in the condition of your hair in as little as a week.

The emotional states associated with the hair, sadness and grief (see chart, page 29), also have a profound effect on the condition of your hair and scalp. When I first met Phyllis, she had a halo of soft, curly blond hair that absolutely shone. I saw her almost every day, since she worked in the coffee shop across the street from my spa. After about a year, however, she moved to Florida because her elderly parents had become ill and needed her care. Several months after she left New York, Phyllis came back for a visit and stopped in to say hello. I was startled by the drastic change in her appearance—especially her hair. Once thick and healthy, it was now thin, lifeless, and gray. She had lost so much hair I could see her scalp at the crown.

When she told me that her mother had died and her father had moved into a nursing home, I understood what had happened to her: the intense sadness and grief over her parents had altered the state of her hair and skin. I didn't know Phyllis well enough to volunteer suggestions that would stop this problem, but had things been different, I would have suggested that she begin by eating foods that would restore balance to her body and ultimately her emotional state.

FOOD FOR FABULOUS HAIR

As with all aspects of our outer beauty, the place to start on the *Tao* to beautiful hair is diet. According to Chinese teaching, healthy kidneys and lungs are the foundations of beautiful hair. If your hair is dull, lifeless, thin, or prone to premature graying, your kidneys may not be functioning optimally, or your *chi* may be off balance. Instead of experimenting with endless shampoos and treatments to bring about healthy, shining hair, you need to restore the balance of your blood *chi*. If you've begun to follow the detoxification and nutritional suggestions in Chapter 4, you may already be seeing some improvement in the condition of your hair and scalp.

I have not broken this chapter down into sections specifically for normal, dry, or oily hair, dandruff, split ends, premature graying, or hair loss. All of these problems—except for overprocessing and chemical damage—stem from the same source: the body's state of imbalance.

A general regimen of kidney-friendly foods and herbs is the first step to rejuvenated, resplendent hair. If the kidneys are healthy, then the lungs and large intestine are healthy . . . and the hair will show it.

Listed below are foods we should all include in our diets.

FOODS FOR HEALTHY HAIR AND SCALP

Fruits and nuts: blackberries, chestnuts, Chinese red and black dates, grapes, papayas, plums, tangerines, walnuts.

Vegetables: black and yellow soybeans, carrots, celery, chives, fennel, ginger, green beans, onions, parsnips, pumpkins, red beans, seaweed (especially arame and hijiki), spinach, sweet potatoes, winter squashes.

Grains and seeds: black sesame seeds, oats, sweet rice, brown rice, whole wheat.

Proteins: chicken, clams, duck, eggs, kidneys, lamb, oysters, white-meat fish.

Miscellaneous: Chinese parsley (coriander) or curly parsley, cinnamon bark, cloves, dang quai, ginseng, licorice root, safflower, wolfberries.

FOODS TO AVOID

Iced or very cold foods and drinks, sugary foods and drinks, colas, coffee, caffeine, fatty foods, red meats, citrus fruits, millet, cheese, milk and other dairy products.

WHERE TO BEGIN

Following are some tips for great hair:

- A mineral-rich multivitamin supplement every day will help strengthen your hair and promote growth. It will also encourage pigment retention.
- Give your hair and scalp a papaya "facial" by peeling and seeding a medium papaya and pureeing it in a blender. Massage this into your hair and scalp and wrap your head in plastic wrap. Cover it with a shower cap or wrap it in a towel. Leave the puree on for fifteen minutes, then wash hair with warm water and a gentle shampoo.
- Treat light brown, blond, or red hair with a lemon juice rinse to bring out the highlights and restore the hair's acid mantle: Mix the juice of one lemon with water—one part lemon juice to five parts water—and use it as a finishing rinse.
- Another great conditioning rinse for blond hair is a cup of strong chamomile tea with a teaspoon of apple cider vinegar.
- Bring out highlights in dark hair by using a cup of strong black tea as a finishing rinse. Like the lemon juice rinse, the tannic acid in the tea restores that all-important acid mantle to your hair.
- Wash your brush and comb every time you wash your hair. If you don't, you'll be brushing and combing oils and dirt back into your freshly washed hair and onto your scalp.
- Never, ever brush your hair when it's wet. Always use a comb with large, rounded teeth to keep from damaging the hair shaft.
- Wear hats and scarves to protect your hair in extreme weather conditions.

RECIPES FOR HEALTHY HAIR AND SCALP

Before getting into the edible recipes that nourish your hair and scalp, here are several recipes that you can use topically to help normalize or balance the condition of your hair and scalp. I'm sure you'll want to add them to your home-spa beauty program.

Heavenly Hair and Scalp Massage Oil   (yin)

A healthy scalp, not to mention a stunning head of hair, is at your fingertips. When we stimulate the circulation in our scalp, our hair follicles thrive from the added nutrients obtained with the increased blood flow. The essential oils in this recipe also loosen dead cells and remove sebaceous oils that clog your pores, so that new hair can grow thick and healthy. Use this oil nightly for a week to stimulate growth, and weekly after that. Repeat this program every six to eight weeks.

Makes one week's supply, enough for 7 treatments

> 1 lemon
> 2 ounces oil of rosemary (see NOTE)
> 1 ounce oil of lavender (see NOTE)

Juice the lemon and strain out any seeds and pulp. Pour into a cup. Add the oils and stir to blend. Pour into a 4-ounce glass medicine bottle— preferably amber (your pharmacist will sell you an empty bottle with a dropper top for pennies). Store in the refrigerator to prevent deterioration of the lemon juice (which will spoil after about a week).

To use, squirt one dropperful of this mixture into a small glass bowl. Wash your hands, then with your fingertips, massage lightly to distribute the oil all over your scalp. Concentrate on your hairline and any areas where hair may be thinning.

Leave on overnight. Your scalp and hair will absorb most of the oils by the time you have finished massaging it in. However, if you're concerned about ruining your pillows, cover them with a towel. In the morning, wash and style your hair as usual.

NOTE: You can find rosemary and lavender oils at herb shops, some health food stores, and anywhere where aromatherapy products are sold, as well as by mail order from the Resources listed on page 253.

Dandruff-Fighting Scalp Tonic   *(yin/yang)*

If you're plagued by a flaky scalp, try this dandruff-fighting tonic. Used weekly, your hair will shimmer and your scalp will be clean. Don't worry about leaving it on overnight—you really won't *smell of vinegar.*

Makes 1 treatment

> ¼ cup apple cider vinegar
> ¼ cup vodka

Mix liquids in a 2-cup measuring cup. Apply liberally with cotton balls to your scalp and the hair close to your scalp, especially if your hair is long. Massage it in with your fingertips to stimulate circulation and distribute the tonic.

Leave on your hair overnight. Wash and style as usual the following morning. Use as a weekly treatment to prevent dandruff, more frequently to cure it.

Flaxseed Styling Gel   *(yin/yang)*

If you've ever had problems with styling products that are too drying or too sticky for your hair, you can make your own for pennies and have something that is gentle, nondrying, and the right consistency for your hair and style. This will keep up to two weeks in the refrigerator.

Makes about 1½ cups

> ¼ cup flaxseed (see NOTE)

Bring 2 cups of water to a rolling boil in a glass or enamel saucepan. Stir in the flax seeds. Reduce heat to simmer and let cook for 10 to 15 minutes, until you have a viscous liquid (the consistency of mucilage). Strain through a fine sieve and discard the seeds.

Return the liquid to a simmer, reducing it to the appropriate consistency for your hair and style. The more you simmer, the stronger the hold your gel will have. Store the gel in a bottle with a tight cap and refrigerate until ready to use.

To use, pour a little into your palms and work into your hair, taking care that you don't let it puddle on your scalp. Comb the gel through to the end of the hair shafts. Style as usual.

NOTE: Flaxseed is readily available in herb shops and health food stores across the country.

ABOUT SHAMPOOS, CONDITIONERS, AND STYLING PRODUCTS

While there are many recipes for homemade shampoos, conditioners, and styling products, I don't know of too many people who will take the time and trouble to make them—especially since there are so many excellent hair products on the market. Store-bought products will do the job as well, and often better, than the home-brewed potions, and they can be far more economical. The oils—basil, bergamot, nettle, rosemary, and lavender, for example—that add fragrance, nutrients, body, and gentle astringence can be costly, and if they are not refrigerated or stored properly, quickly become rancid and lose their potency.

So, instead of asking you to stew and brew and mix and blend batches of things you may use only once, let me give you some guidelines to follow when selecting hair products:

- Buy products that clearly state that they are pH-balanced to protect the acid mantle of the hair and scalp.
- Avoid products that have a high isopropyl or ethyl alcohol content. They are too drying, regardless of the condition of your hair and scalp.
- If you have the slightest question about the hair care you need, ask questions. Ask your stylist, your dermatologist. Call the toll-free numbers listed on product packaging. Ask friends who have great hair what they do to keep it that way. Just do your research until you have answers that make sense to you.

EAT YOUR WAY TO GREAT HAIR

To the Chinese, soup is always the first step to good health. It helps in both the prevention of illness and the healing process. Because our bodies contain mostly water, the vitamins and nutrients in soups are more easily (and immediately) absorbed than from any other food source. In Chinese culture, children are sometimes allowed to skip meals, but they must always drink their soup! And it goes without saying that I am talking about freshly prepared soup with an irresistible aroma that wafts through the house.

Red Beans with Ribs Soup (yin/yang)

This is my all-time favorite soup. In addition to making an appetizing meal, it helps brighten the hair and promote growth. Considered a blood tonic, this popular soup is known for its ability to strengthen the spleen, stomach, and liver. Its ingredients are proven to retard graying and help promote hair growth.

Makes 4 main-dish servings

> 1 cup dried adzuki or kidney beans (see NOTE)
> ¼-inch piece dried tangerine peel (see NOTE)
> 1 large carrot, chopped into ¼-inch pieces
> 1 large onion, coarsely chopped
> 2 stalks celery, cut into 1-inch pieces
> 1 pound lean pork ribs or pork loin, cut into 1-inch pieces
> ½ cup chopped Chinese parsley
> Salt and pepper to taste

Wash the beans and cover with hot water in a large glass bowl; soak for 30 to 45 minutes. Wash the tangerine peel and soak in warm water until ready to use.

Bring 8 cups of water to a boil in a 2-quart enamel soup pot. Add the drained beans and tangerine peel, carrot, onion, celery, pork, and parsley to the boiling water; return to a rolling boil. Reduce heat to medium, cover and simmer for 1 hour, stirring occasionally to prevent sticking, or until the red beans begin to fall apart. Season with salt and pepper.

NOTE: You can use canned beans if desired, as long as they are not pre-seasoned. If using canned beans, wait until pork and vegetables are slightly tender before adding to the soup. Continue cooking for ½ hour. Dried tangerine peel is available at Asian markets and health food stores.

Walnut Chicken with Wolfberries   (yang)

When I was a young girl, this was one of my favorite meals. It wasn't until I began studying herbs and traditional Chinese medicine that I found out this recipe has special ingredients that enhance kidney function and strengthen the eyes. It also promotes lustrous, healthy hair!

Makes 2 to 4 main-dish servings

> 3 to 4 tablespoons corn or vegetable oil
> 1 cup walnut halves
> 1 pound boneless, skinless chicken breast, sliced into ½-inch pieces
> 1½-inch piece ginger, peeled and chopped
> 2 cloves garlic, peeled and chopped
> 2 scallions, cut into small pieces
> ½ cup dried wolfberries, soaked for 20 minutes (see NOTE)
> Salt to taste
>
> *Seasoning Mix*
> 1 teaspoon sugar
> ½ teaspoon finely ground white pepper
> 1 tablespoon soy sauce
> 1 teaspoon sesame oil
> 1 teaspoon cornstarch

Heat 1 tablespoon cooking oil in a wok or skillet. Stir-fry the walnuts for

1 to 2 minutes, until golden brown. Remove from pan and spread on paper towels to drain.

Combine the ingredients for the Seasoning Mix in a glass measuring cup, stirring until the cornstarch is dissolved. Pour over the chicken pieces, and toss to coat. Cover the bowl with plastic wrap and set aside. Allow chicken to marinate at room temperature for 10 minutes, or refrigerated for 20 minutes.

Heat remaining 2 to 3 tablespoons oil in wok or skillet. Quickly stir-fry the ginger, garlic, and scallions. Drain the water from the wolfberries. Discard the water and add the wolfberries to the wok. Then add the chicken—a little at a time—and stir-fry for 3 to 5 minutes, until chicken is white and tender. Season with salt as desired. Add stir-fried walnuts and toss gently to mix.

Serve with rice, if desired.

NOTE: Dried wolfberries are available in Asian markets and from the mail-order Resources listed on page 253.

Walnut-Lamb Stew *(yang)*

Walnuts help tone the kidneys, the main organ that helps us stay youthful. According to Chinese herbal tradition, walnuts also keep the hair and scalp healthy and retard graying. Longan is a Chinese fruit that is dried to use in cooking. When fresh, longans look much like lychees, only smaller and rounder with a smooth tan shell.

Makes 4 to 5 main-dish servings

2 tablespoons (about 12 pieces) dried longans, soaked in warm water
    for 20 minutes; drained (see NOTE)
1-inch piece of ginger, peeled and cut into ¼-inch pieces
½ pound lean lamb stew meat, cut into 1-inch pieces
2 to 3 cloves garlic, peeled and chopped
½ teaspoon ground cloves
¼ teaspoon ground cinnamon
1 cup walnut halves
Soy sauce to taste
Pepper to taste

Place all ingredients except soy sauce and pepper in a 2-quart enamel saucepan with lid. Add 6 to 8 cups of water, bring to a boil, and stir. Reduce heat to medium and cover. Simmer for 45 minutes to an hour, until meat and longans are tender. Season with soy sauce and pepper to taste.

NOTE: Dried longans are available from Asian markets and from the mail-order Resources listed on page 253.

Peanut-Seaweed Soup   (yin/yang)

Lustrous, manageable hair will be just one of the benefits of this tasty soup. It helps improve digestion by bringing balance to the stomach and spleen, while promoting good chi and kidney energy.

Makes 4 to 5 main-dish servings

  ⅓ cup shelled raw peanuts with skins, washed and soaked
      overnight (leave skins on)
  1 pound lean pork ribs or pork loin, cut into 1-inch cubes
  2 or 3 sheets or strips of seaweed (kelp or kombu), broken into
      small pieces
  ¼-inch piece dried mandarin orange peel, soaked in hot water
      for 2 to 3 minutes (see NOTE)
  1-inch piece ginger, cut into ¼-inch pieces
  Salt and pepper to taste

Place all ingredients except salt and pepper in a 4-quart enamel soup pot with lid. Add 8 cups of water, bring to a boil, then simmer on low-medium heat for 1 hour, or until the pork is cooked through and peanuts are soft. Add salt and pepper to taste.

NOTE: Dried mandarin peel is available at Asian markets and health food stores.

Black Sesame Seed Soup *(yin/yang)*

This soup is so sweet that my family enjoys it for dessert or as a snack. It's as sweet as ice cream, and ever so much more healthful. It can be easily reheated and can be enjoyed at any time of day. Long-term consumption of this treat beautifies the scalp and hair as well as the skin.

Makes two 1-cup servings

> 1 cup uncooked long-grain white rice
> 1 cup black sesame seeds
> 1 tablespoon sugar, or to taste

Wash and drain the rice and the sesame seeds in separate containers. Stir-fry the sesame seeds in a dry skillet over low heat for 5 minutes, or until the heat releases their fragrance. Don't let them burn.

Grind the rice and toasted seeds with ¼ cup water in a blender. Pour this mixture plus 1¾ cups water into a medium-size saucepan, and cook over medium heat for 10 minutes, stirring often to avoid burning. Add the sugar as desired.

7.

SPECIAL CARE FOR
YOUR HANDS, FEET, AND NAILS

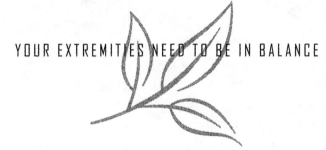

YOUR EXTREMITIES NEED TO BE IN BALANCE

The Chinese believe that the hands and feet require care that goes beyond mere manicures, pedicures, hand lotion, and pumice stones. The same yin/yang balance applied to all other aspects of the Organic Whole applies here as well. To keep those elements in focus, maintaining equilibrium, is always the essential goal. You will find that, consciously applied, this philosophy is easy to work into your lifestyle and will benefit each part of your body.

Centuries of research show that the condition of the hands and feet can be altered and even corrected by restoring balance to the systems of the body. In the Tao of beauty, the hands and feet—like the ear—represent a microcosm of the entire body. Acupuncture and acupressure were developed just for this reason—practitioners see the hands and feet as maps, with certain areas on each corresponding to organs in the body. The toes, for example, reflect the conditions of the sinuses and head—left and right, depending on the foot being treated. The inside line of the foot, from the big toe to the heel, reflects the spine, from the head and neck to the coccyx. When pressure is applied, stagnant *chi* is released so that healing energy can flow to the corresponding organs.

THE HANDS TELL ALL

Everybody notices hands. The rough, strong hands of a laborer; the callused yet pliant fingertips of a guitarist; the strong, supple hands of a massage therapist—all speak volumes not only about one's profession but about one's self-image. Gnawed cuticles and stubby nails with chipped polish hardly reflect high self-esteem. According to Chinese lore, the hands are the "gates to Paradise," no doubt because of their ability to touch and move, and are considered the ultimate indicator of a woman's femininity. Early Chinese doctors reasoned that smooth, supple hands and strong, evenly shaped fingernails indicated a healthy, balanced body; pale, stiff hands and uneven, weak nails reflected stagnant *chi* function not just in the hands and fingers but throughout the entire body.

During one of the winter collection shows in Milan, a model friend named Debbie commented that I had nice hands and nails. Her nails, she complained, seemed to never grow. Because they were so stubby, Debbie was ashamed to have her nails done professionally. When necessary for a specific modeling assignment, she would glue on fake nails or, if appropriate, wear gloves or carry a scarf or some other accessory to deflect attention away from her fingers.

I told Debbie that if she really wanted better-looking hands and nails, the first thing she should do was get a professional manicure. A good manicurist would shape her nails correctly and push the cuticles back. This would create the illusion of longer, neater nails and stimulate nail growth. Even more important, she would get a great hand massage. Everything a manicurist does encourages the flow of blood and *chi* energy to and from the extremities, which is essential to beautiful hands and nails.

I also suggested that since her schedule was so chaotic, she should learn to give herself a manicure. I told her to brush her nails with a natural-bristle nail brush and mild soap during her bath or shower to help get rid of dead cuticle cells. And I suggested that she massage her fingertips and cuticles every night with a moisturizing cream or even petroleum jelly. This would stimulate her circulation while strengthening and rehydrating the nail beds. Nails lose moisture twice as fast as skin, mainly because they are less porous and less absorbent. Our hands are exposed to a great deal of water, often without being properly dried. By applying a thick, topical ointment such as lanolin or petroleum jelly to your nails and cuticles, you can virtually eliminate hangnails, ingrown toenails, and dry nails and cuticles. There are several fine nail creams on the market, but lanolin or petroleum jelly do the same job for much less money.

Of course, I gave Debbie a list of foods she should include in her diet: grapes, peaches, plums, asparagus, snow peas, tofu, white-fleshed fish, shrimp, brown rice, and more. These foods, and others listed on page 146, increase the flow of *chi* in addition to balancing the hot and cold energy throughout the body.

When the next show season came around, I noticed that Debbie had gorgeous nails. She thanked me profusely and said that she couldn't have had them without me!

WHAT YOUR HANDS SAY ABOUT YOU

Undeniably, hands reflect a person's state of health. A traditional Chinese practitioner looks for signs that indicate a variety of conditions, most of which can be corrected by restoring balance to the entire body. Following are a few common hand conditions and what they may say about you:

- Hot, even warm, hands can indicate excess internal heat. Other signs of this yang condition are dry, scaly, or red skin. Increasing the moisture of the yin organs, especially the kidneys, is recommended. This is usually done with herbal teas, cooling mint or green tea for example, and juices—apple, grapefruit, and grape will do. Ginger and orange peel, either together or separately, are especially effective for bringing balance to this condition, despite their individual yang properties.
- Hands that are cold and pale can indicate excessive internal cold and stagnant *chi*. Replenishing the yang organs, especially the yang energy of the kidneys is vital. Dang quai and Chinese licorice, taken either together or separately in a tea, are particularly helpful for this. See the food list on

pages 46–47 and incorporate foods from the yang list into your diet to increase internal warming.

- Clammy hands indicate too much dampness or moisture in the system, as well as in the atmosphere. In some people this shows up as arthritis; in others, merely as occasional twinges of pain in the joints. Feeding the yang energy of the spleen and lungs will help correct this. The traditional drink given to old people with pain in the joints of their hands and feet is a tea of astragalus, Chinese cinnamon, ginger, Paeonia, and Chinese red dates. You'll find out more about arthritis later in this chapter.

These problems show up not only in the hands. They also manifest themselves in the feet. Therefore, any treatment that promotes the health of the hands is, in all probability, applicable to the feet.

FANCY FOOTWORK

Feet are even more complex than hands in terms of their relationship to the rest of the body. They have the responsibility of bearing our weight and maintaining balance as we move from place to place. Even the slightest pain in the foot can radiate throughout your body, affecting posture and otherwise throwing your body out of balance. Since our feet are our most abused body parts, it is wise to take special care of them. The great Chinese warrior Sun Ye said it best several thousands years ago when he wrote that "the strength of an army is only as good as one soldier's feet."

Take care to examine your feet closely, not just around the nails, but all over. Use a mirror if you must, but look at the soles and peek between your toes for any indication of cuts or fungal growth. Examine your heels, and look especially at your instep and ankles. Cuts and bruises on the feet can take a long time to heal. Diminished circulation, moisture, heat from wearing closed, unvented shoes, wearing shoes that don't fit properly, or even the pressure of holding your body upright can create conditions that may lead to complications, including fungus, thickened skin, rough spots on the heels and balls of your feet, as well as bone deformities.

Be very careful when cutting your toenails. Cut them straight across and never down into the corners. If you do, you may develop ingrown toenails, especially on your big toes. Each time you do this, the nail will grow deeper, which can lead to myriad problems.

WHAT YOUR NAILS SAY ABOUT YOU

The condition of your nails—be they on your fingers or your toes—provides a major clue to the condition of your body and, in the big picture, your beauty. No matter what polish colors them, healthy nails are always strong and smooth, with a clear, rosy pink nail bed and smooth, pliable cuticle. This indicates that you have ample blood production and circulation, that your *chi* flows uninhibited throughout your body.

When the nail bed is pale or discolored, you may have insufficient blood production, and your circulation of blood and energy may be slow. Ridged or grooved nails tell a traditional Chinese practitioner that you may be experiencing imbalances in your liver. This can mean a problem with calcium absorption, which inhibits bone development. Poor blood circulation and calcium depletion point directly to deficiencies in the wood element and the organs associated with it—the liver and gallbladder. Therefore it's important to include foods in your diet that nourish these organs.

Healthy nails are not ridged, nor are they speckled with white spots. They are not brittle, do not flake in layers, and do not break easily. These conditions are all indicators of inadequate or stagnant liver *chi*. Thickened nails or nails that are separated from the bed may indicate the presence of fungus or infection in the system. Bringing all systems of the body into balance ultimately eradicates these conditions.

Manicures and pedicures make your hands and feet feel great and *appear* better, which hopefully inspires you to take better care of them. However, you must nurture them from within by including plenty of water, healthy foods, teas, and herbal recipes to provide the appropriate cold or hot energy and nutrients to the organs involved.

FOODS FOR HEALTHY HANDS, FEET, AND NAILS

Fruits and nuts: blackberries, chestnuts, Chinese red and black dates, papayas, peaches, pears, pumpkins, red grapes, strawberries, tangerines, walnuts, water chestnuts.

Vegetables: asparagus, black and yellow soybeans, broccoli, carrots, celery, Chinese cabbage (bok choy), chives, collards, fennel, green beans, kale, mushrooms, onions, parsnips, pinto and other red beans, snow peas, spinach, sword beans, tofu, tomatoes, watercress, winter squash.

Grains and seeds: barley, black sesame seeds, brown rice, corn, oats, wheat gluten, whole wheat.

Proteins: chicken, crab (especially soft shell crab), duck, kidneys, lamb, pork, oysters, oxtails, shrimp, white-fleshed fish, meat tendons, shark fins, meat or fish bones for making soup.

Herbs and spices: Chinese licorice root, Chinese parsley (coriander), chives, cinnamon bark, cloves, dang quai, garlic (raw), ginger, ginseng, curly-leafed parsley, sea cucumber, wheatgrass, wolfberries.

FOODS TO AVOID

Cheese, citrus fruits, nuts and nut butters (except walnuts), salt (use only in moderation), processed sugar, sugary foods and drinks, red meats.

WHAT YOU CAN DO FOR BEAUTIFUL HANDS AND FEET

Besides incorporating the right foods into your diet, there are other things you can do to beautify your hands and feet. Take special care of your extremities so that you can repair any damage and prevent more from occurring. Here's how:

- Since your hands are often the first place to show your age, make it a habit to give them a massage with a rich moisturizing product as part of your nightly bedtime routine. If possible, buy a moisturizer made from natural ingredients (jojoba oil, lanolin, etc.) and use it often. Moisturize and massage your feet too, at bedtime.

- By massaging cream into your hands and fingertips, feet and toes, you stimulate pressure points that release tension all over your body. This leaves not only your hands and feet feeling refreshed and rejuvenated but the rest of your body as well. Even if it's just for a couple of minutes as you dry off after bathing, massage sends the flow of blood and stagnant *chi* from the toes back into circulation.
- After massaging creams and lotions into your hands and feet, slip on white cotton gloves and socks and wear them through the night. This will keep your hands and feet soft, and your nails moist, strong, and pliable.
- Always rub your hands with a moisturizing cream and wear thin white cotton gloves before exercising, especially if you are going to be outdoors. This will help the skin retain moisture. Sun, wind, and airborne pollutants can do serious damage to tender skin. And don't forget sunscreen on the backs of your hands and tops of your feet whenever they are exposed.
- Rub white iodine into your fingernails and toenails with cotton balls to strengthen your nails (regular iodine will leave a rather unattractive stain). I recommend doing this nightly for a week or two until your nails are stronger. Do it weekly after that.
- Always wear gloves when doing chores, indoors and out. Fabric-lined rubber gloves are a *must* for any task that involves water or chemicals. Heavy canvas gloves are essential for gardening—even working with your houseplants. Soft cotton gloves are enough for almost everything else— sweeping, vacuuming, making beds.
- After your bath or shower, gently erase rough spots and calluses on your heels and soles with a damp pumice stone. This will keep your feet smooth and less prone to injury.
- Keep your feet dry. Moisture makes mayhem with your feet. Wear vented shoes or, if that's not possible, take off your shoes several times during the day to allow them to breathe and dry. Perspiration is vital to the body's temperature-regulating system as well as to elimination of body wastes, but wear stockings or socks to absorb any moisture that may collect in your shoes.
- Eliminate swelling and improve circulation by alternating hot and cold

soaks. Fill one deep pan with hot water and Epsom salts and another with cold water and ice cubes. Dip your feet in the hot water for two minutes to dilate veins and capillaries, then move to the iced water for two minutes. Repeat this process, moving from hot to cold, for ten minutes. If your ankles are especially swollen, use a ladle to pour hot and then cold water on your shins and calves.

- Drink plenty of water to keep your kidneys flushed with fluid. This helps to prevent water retention in your feet and hands.
- Stand and place your hands against a wall for balance. Place a small hard rubber ball (or a tennis ball) on the floor. Roll the ball under one foot and then the other. Make sure that you flex your ankles and stretch your toes over the ball. Roll it under the ball of your foot as you press into it, then slide the ball under the arch and work it back so that you can roll your heel over it. Take your foot off the ball and stand up straight, away from the wall. Feel how much looser and more energized that side of your body is? Repeat with the other foot. Do this several times a day to keep your *chi* moving.

MODEL HANDS

While most models work at fashion shows and photo shoots for fashion layouts and advertisements, some are specialists like Jean. She is a hand model. You've probably seen her hands in magazines and on television, holding a bottle of laundry detergent or luxurious perfume, modeling a wedding band or bracelet, displaying the latest nail enamel colors. Her face rarely shows, so you probably wouldn't even suspect that she is a model, especially since she is considerably shorter than the five-foot-nine minimum height required for fashion modeling. Her hands are absolutely beautiful, exquisitely shaped, with amazing fingernails. There's not a flaw, blemish, or wrinkle on them.

When we met, I was so impressed that I couldn't help myself. I blurted right out, "I'll bet you haven't washed a dish or touched a mop in years!"

Quite the contrary. Jean assured me that she does indeed wash dishes. The big difference is that she wears gloves, no matter what she is doing—cotton-lined rubber gloves for tasks that involve water, cotton gloves for dusting and vacuuming, canvas work gloves in the garden. She also uses real tools, instead of her fingernails, for every task. You'd never catch *her* scratching candle wax off the dining table with her thumbnail!

There are also foot models who treat their feet with rigorous care. They never go barefoot, unless for a photo shoot, and they always wear shoes that fit. You'll never find them squeezing their size 9½ tootsies into size 9 pumps, or slopping around in last season's stretched-out sandals.

All of this is to say that you can do almost anything, as long as you take precautions and make adjustments in *how* you perform tasks to prevent damage. Like everything else in life, balance in our behavior, like balance in our meals, is the key.

WATER WORKS . . . AND OTHER HANDY TRICKS

Lack of fluids and moisture in our diets and our bodies can leave us with dry, chapped hands and feet and unhealthy fingernails. Refer back to Chapter 5, especially to the recipes for dry skin, and incorporate them into your diet and skin-care regimen.

Water is the best natural diuretic in the world. If you are the least bit prone to fluid retention, especially in your hands, feet, or ankles, increase your water intake from six to eight glasses of water to eight to ten glasses, and cut your consumption of salty and fatty foods by half.

Avoid developing enlarged veins in your hands at all costs. This is a dead giveaway of age. Avoid carrying heavy packages. When you carry a shopping bag that is light, there is no problem. However, if it is heavy, you have to use a lot of strength, causing blood to flow into your hands and becoming trapped in your fingers. When you hold tightly onto the handles of shopping bags, this can interrupt circulation considerably, especially if you carry these packages down by your sides. Blood builds up and enlarges the veins. I suggest using a shopping cart or, if that's not possible, putting the parcels down at frequent intervals and holding your hands over your head to restore circulation. I hold my hands high and, when possible, carry things above my waist. I know this looks a little odd, so in public I gently cross my arms while keeping my fingertips up. No one even suspects I'm saving my hands.

I'm not the first woman to wave her hands over her head in the name of beauty. I am told that Marilyn Monroe held her arms over her head and wiggled her hands around to reduce swelling before stepping onto the set.

ABOUT ARTHRITIS

The Chinese name for this painful condition is *fung sup quat tong* which literally means "wet wind, bone pain." These two phrases go together, as one always follows the other.

Because women, more often than men, still do most of the cooking and cleanup, and as a consequence have their hands in and out of water, women experience arthritis in their hands more often than men do.

We know that water and air are cooling properties, which are often used to alleviate other imbalances in the hands and feet. Such chilled energy, however, can result in blocked energy flow and slowed blood circulation that affects your bones and joints. People with arthritis suffer most on cold or rainy days.

The Chinese also believe that arthritis can be inherited from our ancestors. If our ancestors worked with their hands, kept them in water, and then developed arthritis, this condition could pass on to you. If you treat your hands the same way, you risk passing arthritis on to your offspring. This is another good reason to take care of your hands and joints.

An important way to prevent arthritis is to dry your hands thoroughly after washing them or getting them wet. Always wear fabric-lined rubber gloves when washing dishes, and wear disposable latex gloves—like your doctor or dentist or the cook at your corner diner uses—to protect your hands while cooking. Gloves provide protection for your skin and manicure without limiting movement. Remember to apply moisturizing lotion before donning the gloves. Take care to wash and rinse gloves thoroughly before handling food to remove any detergent residue. Also wash gloves thoroughly after using them, and make sure that they are dry on the inside before using them again. Throw away the disposables.

RECIPES FOR HEALTHY HANDS AND FEET

These recipes for hand and foot treatments and delicious dishes use ingredients that are known to provide the energy and nutrients necessary for healthy, beautiful hands, feet, and nails. Look back to Chapter 5 for other topical skin recipes you'll want to use (for dry skin for example).

Ginger-Licorice Hand and Foot Soak (yang)

Ginger and licorice have amazing properties that contribute to the health and beauty of your hands and feet. Ginger stimulates circulation of both blood and chi. This brings a warming energy that helps to remove coldness, aches, swelling, and numbness. Chinese licorice is widely recognized for its fungicidal properties, which protect your nails and feet from the often-painful problems of nail fungus and athlete's foot.

Makes 1 soak

> 8 to 12 ounces ginger, cut into long strips
> 6 to 8 slices Chinese licorice root (see NOTE)

Pound the ginger with a mallet to break up the fibers. Pound the licorice roots lightly to release essence.

Boil the ginger and licorice with 6 cups of water in a glass or enamel saucepan for 5 to 10 minutes, until liquid is the color of weak tea.

Strain, reserving liquid, and let cool slightly. Soak hands and/or feet in this warm solution for 10 to 15 minutes, until water is tepid. Dry hands and/or feet thoroughly with a soft towel.

NOTE: Chinese licorice root has healing properties not found in American-grown roots. You can purchase it in Asian markets and many larger health food stores as well as from the mail-order Resources listed on page 253.

Journey-of-a-Thousand-Miles Foot Sparkle   (yin/yang)

A wise man once said, "A journey of a thousand miles begins with a single step." Easier said than done, if your feet are sore! As a model, I found that after ten hour days of strutting up and down the catwalk in stiletto heels, my feet ached for hours. I invented this footbath for my friends and myself when we needed to get back on our feet. It is relaxing, detoxifying, and combats stagnant chi.

Makes 2 footbaths (16 ounces)

> 10 nonbuffered adult-strength aspirin
> ¼ cup baking soda
> ¼ cup Epsom salts
> 10 drops oil of peppermint (see NOTE)
> 5 drops oil of spearmint (see NOTE)
> 5 drops oil of wintergreen (see NOTE)
> 5 drops oil of eucalyptus (see NOTE)

Crush aspirin in a large glass bowl. Mix the baking soda and Epsom salts with the crushed aspirin. Add the essential oils and mix until the oils are thoroughly incorporated into the mixture.

Pour the salt mixture onto a clean flat surface, such as a cookie sheet, and place in a warm, dry place overnight. Do not cover. Stir to make certain mixture is dry. If not, let it sit another day. If your climate is too humid for the salts and oils to air-dry, place in a 200°F oven and bake for 15 minutes. Do not microwave. Pour into a clean, airtight container—preferably glass. Store tightly closed in a dry place.

To use: Dissolve half of this mixture in a pan of hot water. Soak your feet for 15 to 20 minutes. Dry feet thoroughly after using. Do not reuse soaking water.

NOTE: These oils are available in herb shops and many health food stores. You can also purchase them in some specialty or natural pharmacies or from the mail-order Resources listed on page 253.

Fantastic Footsteps Softening Treatment   (yin/yang)

Another sensational way to soften your feet and remove those ugly calluses is to use this easy-to-make softening treatment. The acids in the fruits work wonders on dry, thickened skin, while the pepper and vinegar stimulate the flow of chi.

Makes 1 treatment

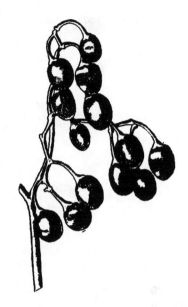

> 1 medium ripe papaya, peeled
> 1 cup canned crushed pineapple, with juice
> 1 teaspoon cayenne pepper
> 2 tablespoons kosher salt
> 1 tablespoon white vinegar

Wolfberries (*Solanum dulcamara*)

Place papaya—seeds and skin as well as fruit—and the pineapple in a blender. Add the cayenne, kosher salt, and vinegar. Process until thoroughly pureed.

Divide this mixture equally into two plastic bags. Stick your feet into the bags and squish them around so that your feet are covered. Place towels over your feet to prevent leakage.

Sit quietly for 20 minutes. Lift one foot from the bag and massage gently, using the crushed papaya seeds and salt to remove roughness. Rinse thoroughly, first under warm water, then under cold, to increase circulation. Repeat with the other foot.

Wolfberry Tea   (yin/yang)

You may not have heard of wolfberries before, but you'll make sure that you keep them on hand after this. These tiny, sweet berries are orange to red in color, depending on the region of China where they are grown. They are known to bring warming energy to the liver, gallbladder, and kidneys—which means they're good for lots of things, from arthritis to clear eyes to dry skin. Most Chinese households use them regularly in soups and teas . . . and even soak them in wine.

Makes 2 servings

> 2 to 3 tablespoons dried wolfberries (see NOTE)
> Honey to taste

Place water and wolfberries in a glass or enamel saucepan; bring to a boil. Stir to mix, then cover and reduce heat. Simmer over low heat for 5 minutes. Taste and sweeten with honey if desired.

NOTE: You can purchase dried wolfberries in health food stores and Asian markets, as well as from the mail-order Resources listed on page 253.

Honey Soybean Milk   *(yin)*

This nutritious high-protein drink is a beauty must for your nails. The honey provides antiseptic and moisturizing properties that also make your hair shiny and your skin soft.

Makes 1 cup

> 1 cup soy milk
> 1 teaspoon honey

Heat soy milk in a glass or enamel saucepan. Sweeten with honey to taste. Drink once a day for a week and notice the difference in the strength and color of your nails.

Black Soybean Soup   (yin/yang)

If you suffer from arthritis, you'll want to try this hearty soup. Black soybeans encourage the circulation of blood and other body fluids, helping to relieve the swelling and joint pain associated with arthritis. The beans and fish also serve to nurture the kidneys, stimulating the flow of chi *throughout the body.*

Makes 4 to 6 main-dish servings

> 1 cup dried black soybeans, washed and soaked in water overnight
> in a covered glass bowl (see NOTE)
> 1 pound carp or sea bass fillets, boned and cut into 1-inch cubes
> ½ pound pork loin or lean boneless pork roast, cut into 1-inch cubes
> 2 stalks celery, cut diagonally into ½-inch pieces
> 1 large carrot, peeled and cut diagonally into ½-inch pieces
> 6 to 8 cloves garlic, peeled and crushed
> 1 medium onion, cut into 8 wedges
> 1 bunch parsley, coarsely chopped
> 1½-inch piece ginger, peeled and cut into 3 pieces
> 2 tablespoons soy sauce

Place all ingredients in a 4-quart enamel soup pot. Bring to a rolling boil, stirring occasionally to prevent sticking and to mix ingredients. Reduce heat and cover; simmer over medium heat for 1½ hours, or until beans are tender and pork is thoroughly cooked. Stir occasionally to prevent sticking.

NOTE: Dried black soybeans can be found in most health food stores. If unavailable, you can substitute any dried black bean.

Green and Gold Stir-Fry   (yin/yang)

Vegetarians will enjoy this colorful main dish rich with good things to nourish the bodily systems that benefit your hands and feet. You'll serve this quick and easy stir-fry often.

Makes 2 to 4 main-dish servings

> 2 tablespoons light vegetable oil
> 3 to 5 cloves garlic, peeled and chopped
> 2 cups broccoli florets
> 1 large or 2 medium carrots, sliced into ¼-inch coins
> 4 to 6 scallions, cut into 1-inch pieces
> 8 to 10 button mushrooms, sliced thinly
> 1 cup snow peas or green beans, trimmed of stems
> 2 tablespoons honey
> 3 tablespoons soy sauce

Heat oil in a wok; quickly stir-fry the garlic until golden. Add the broccoli and stir-fry lightly for 1 minute. Add carrots, scallions, mushrooms, and snow peas or beans. Gently stir-fry 1 to 2 minutes. Add ¼ cup water, reduce heat, and cover wok for 2 to 4 minutes, until vegetables are tender. Combine honey and soy sauce in wok; stir to blend. Serve over rice, if desired.

Coconut Shrimp Soup   (yin/yang)

A gourmet meal with health-food properties! This delicately flavored main-dish soup is filled with ingredients that build strong, hard nails—especially shrimp and pork neck bones.

Makes 4 main-dish servings

½ pound medium or large shrimp, cleaned, deveined,
    and shells reserved
¾ pound pork neck bones
1 cup coconut meat, preferably fresh, cut into 1-inch pieces
1½-inch piece ginger, peeled and cut into 3 pieces
½ cup Chinese parsley, coarsely chopped
1 small carrot, peeled and shredded
4 to 6 cloves garlic, peeled and chopped
Juice of 1 lemon
Salt and pepper to taste
1 teaspoon roasted sesame oil, optional

If using large shrimp, split in half, lengthwise. Place shrimp in a glass bowl, cover with plastic wrap, and refrigerate until ready to use. Tie shrimp shells in a muslin or cheesecloth bag and cover with 8 cups of water in a 3- or 4-quart enamel soup pot. Bring to a rolling boil and cook over medium heat for 10 minutes. Remove bag.

Wash pork neck bones and place in a single layer in a roasting pan. Place in a 400°F oven for 10 minutes to render excess fat from the bones.

Drain fat from pork neck bones and add the bones to soup pot. Add coconut meat, ginger, parsley, carrot, and garlic. Cover and reduce heat to medium. Cook for 30 minutes, stirring occasionally. Add shrimp. Continue cooking for 5 to 10 minutes, until shrimp are pink and firm. Stir in lemon juice. Add salt, pepper, and sesame oil if desired.

8.

CAST AN EYE ON BEAUTY

TAKE CARE OF YOUR EYES

An ancient proverb says, "The eyes reflect the inner illumination; the gaze reflects the soul." This holds true in *all* cultures. A woman's eyes are regarded as a true reflection of her inner harmony, her inner beauty. Of all our features, our eyes are the most expressive.

It's no wonder that women collectively spend small fortunes every year on mascara, shadows, and liners, not to mention the miracle creams that promise to remove wrinkles and firm the skin around our eyes. Then, when this "magic in a bottle" fails to deliver as promised, we spend an even larger fortune on surgical procedures to repair the damage caused by life and aging. All this fuss over our eyes, yet we seldom stop to think about the *health* of our eyes.

As a fashion model, I have to admit it: I love makeup. And facials, steams, treatment masks, and massage not only make me feel good, they make me healthy. I'm certain that this delight in the most feminine of all activities influenced my decision to develop the products and programs that have evolved into my day spa. Still, simply using the right makeup and skin-care products to enhance appearance is not enough.

I know that I've said it again and again, but internal well-being really does have everything to do with beauty, even with the beauty and health of our eyes. As I discussed on page 19, all facial senses and features tell a story about what is happening inside us.

TRADITIONAL WISDOM

Almost from the very beginning, traditional Chinese herbalists linked the appearance and condition of the eyes with the functioning of the liver, maintaining that the *chi* of the liver nourishes the eyes. Acupuncturists say that the liver meridian passes straight through the eyes, directly affecting the condition of the eyes. As you know from the chart on page 29, the liver and eyes are both related to the element wood. Western physicians learned that jaundice—when the whites of the eyes appear yellow and the skin takes on a yellow cast—can be traced to liver malfunction.

In most cases, problems affecting our eyes result directly from either excessive hot or yang *chi* or deficient nutrition in the body, particularly in the liver. Common eye conditions include inflammation, pink or red eye, eyestrain, and puffiness around the eyes. In addition to internal malfunctions and imbalances, stress can take a definite toll on our eyes, creating crow's-feet and fine wrinkles. Weakened *chi* in the kidneys and liver interrupts function of these vital organs, resulting in dark circles under the eyes.

Try the following acupressure techniques for eyestrain and resulting headaches:

- Gently massage the acupressure points on both sides of the bridge of your nose, next to your eyes. You may notice that you're already doing this unconsciously when your eyes are tired—this is a simple example of how your body can be sensitive to its needs and directs you, through your intuition, to meet those needs.

- Gently rub the pressure points above the bridge of the nose (the "third eye"), the outside of your eyebrows (next to your temples), and on either side of your spine at the base of your skull. You'll be able to identify these points, as they will feel slightly tender to the touch. Use a steady pressure and rub in small circles.
- Press the thumb and forefinger of one hand into the web between your thumb and forefinger of the other—you'll know that you have the right spot because it will feel a bit tender to the touch. Press steadily and hold for several seconds, then repeat the process, pressing into the web of the other hand.

These are important acupuncture points that stimulate the flow of *chi* throughout the body and release endorphins that ease pain. You can use a drop of aromatic oil—rose or lavender, perhaps—or a massage oil, such as Shiling oil or White Flower oil, as you massage these points. The latter two oils, which are sold in Chinese herbal shops and many health food stores, are mildly camphorated, so take care that you don't use them too close to your eyes. They help speed energy through the body to clear the wind energy that can cause tension and headaches.

THE POWER OF FOODS TO ENHANCE OUR EYES

Whenever there is *anything* wrong with our eyes, we are less than beautiful. And it takes more than a new shade of shadow or under-eye concealer to make everything right. Start by providing your body with nourishment. This brings the liver, as well as the kidneys and gallbladder, into balance. By diet, we can do much to improve the condition of our eyes.

Try to reduce the fat in your diet and limit alcohol consumption to take stress off your liver and encourage the flow of *chi*. You can also reduce liver stress and strengthen both the liver and gallbladder by eating four or five *small* meals a day; stop eating several hours before bedtime to give these organs time to rest and regenerate. Incorporate as many foods for healthy eyes as you can from the following list.

FOODS THAT PROMOTE HEALTHY EYES

Fruits and nuts: apples, blackberries, dates, figs, grapefruits, grapes, lemons, melons, oranges, papayas, pears, pineapples, plums, Chinese red and black dates, tangerines.

Vegetables: adzuki beans, bean sprouts, beet roots and tops, bitter melon (wild cucumbers), broccoli, carrots, celery, chicory, cucumbers, dandelion greens, garlic, ginger, green beans, lentils, black beans, lima beans, lotus root, lotus plumule (the green sprout in the seed), onions, spinach, split peas, water chestnuts, watercress.

Grains and seeds: barley grass and grain, black sesame seeds, brown rice, millet, sweet rice, wheat germ, wheat bran, whole grains.

Proteins: clams, fish (especially low-fat white fish such as cod, haddock, flounder, and scrod), tofu.

Herbs: cinnamon bark, chrysanthemum flowers, honeysuckle flowers, licorice root, Oolong tea, nettles, peppermint, wolfberries.

FOODS TO AVOID

Black and white pepper; cheese and other dairy products; mustard greens; star anise; processed sugars, sugary foods and drinks.

PILLOW TALK

Puffiness around the eyes is a dead giveaway that you're doing something wrong. When I was modeling full-time, flying around the world and working around the clock, I learned several tricks to help solve this problem; the most common trick is to lie on your back for ten minutes with a slice of cucumber over each eye. Many makeup artists kept alcohol-free toner in the fridge with cotton balls at the ready to use as compresses before they worked their wizardry with concealers and toners to make the swelling invisible before the camera or on the catwalk.

Here are some other ways to reduce swelling around the eyes:

- Curtail your intake of water and other liquids at night to help reduce eye puffiness. Yes, water is superimportant to your overall health and beauty, but it is best drunk in the morning and afternoon hours.
- Sleep with a large, fluffy pillow. While any type of pillow—firm, medium, or soft—will do, I prefer a full-loft goose-down pillow. Some of you may want foam instead of feathers; others will simply want a fuller, firmer pillow, in which case a traditional buckwheat pillow is fine. But, in general, the more expensive the pillow the better. Believe me, finding the right pillow is money well spent. Nothing beats a good night's sleep, so it would be wise to consider carefully what pillow you want to buy. After all, we spend more than a third of our lives sleeping, so where we lay our heads is important.
- Make a cup of either chrysanthemum or green tea, let it cool, then dip cotton balls into the tea and place them on your eyes. Both chrysanthemum and green tea help rest the eyes and reduce puffiness.

I remembered some things my mother always did to make sure that she awoke refreshed and relaxed . . . and decidedly not puffy. My favorite—and probably the most effective—of these measures is the herbal pillow. These pillows have been used in China since ancient times, and I recommend them highly!

Here's how to make your own:

Chrysanthemum Flower Pillow

These fragrant blooms are known to provide energy to the liver, helping the flow of chi. Chrysanthemum is also known to improve vision, decrease puffiness around the eyes, help blurred vision, and even lower your blood pressure! You'll wake up with a clear head and clear eyes. You can also make the pillow with Oolong tea leaves. This aromatic tea is known to help brighten the eyes, deepen sleep, clear the brain, and even cure a hangover. I recommend this highly to anyone who is under a lot of stress. It will help you get a good rest with a short amount of sleep.

Makes 1 pillow

1 pound dried chrysanthemum petals (see NOTE)
2 small (11 by 14-inch) pillow cases, or 1 zippered pillow cover and
    1 pillowcase

Check the flowers to make sure there are no stems and that they do not clump together. Pour the dried flowers into a clean, fresh pillowcase. Smooth out the petals so the pillowcase is even—don't overstuff it or the pillow will be too hard—and either stitch the pillow shut or zip the pillow cover shut. Put the flower-filled bag into another pillowcase that can be washed.

When selecting your cases, be sure that the cotton is thick and tightly woven; you don't want little bits and pieces of flowers in your bed. About every two or three months, open the inner pillow, take out the flowers, and replace them with new, fresh ones. Place inside a clean pillowcase.

You can use this pillow on top of your "real" pillow or roll it up and use it as a neck roll. When you make your bed, slip your herbal pillow under the covers to keep the aroma strong.

NOTE: Dried chrysanthemum petals are available at herb shops and health food stores or from the mail-order Resources listed on page 253.

FOOD FOR YOUR EYES

One of the best foods to eat to detoxify the liver and rebalance its *chi* is bitter melon (also known as wild cucumber). It can be found in any Chinese market and increasingly in gourmet vegetable stores. It is quite bitter, which may make it an acquired taste. Personally, I love it, but most of my Western friends—and even some Chinese—do not. To remove its bitterness, wash and slice the bitter melon and soak it in boiling water for two minutes. Drain and then submerge in cold water. Drain it again and place in a glass bowl. Sprinkle salt over the slices and let them sit for fifteen minutes. Rinse in cold water to remove the salt and drain on a paper towel. You can use bitter melon in salads, soups, or in the popular dish on page 165, Bitter Melon and Beef in Black Bean Sauce.

If bitter melon is not to your liking, ordinary cucumbers can also be helpful in improving your eyesight; they also detoxify the liver. Remember: the liver "rules" the eyes, so the foods and herbs that help the liver will also help your eyes.

To remove the oil in cucumbers that makes them hard to digest for some people, peel and slice the cucumbers and place them in a glass bowl. Cover the cucumbers with ice cubes and pour a quarter cup of salt over the ice. After fifteen minutes, pour off the ice and water, then rinse the cucumbers under cold water to remove excess salt. Drain cucumber slices on paper towels, then toss them into a salad or use them in soups or any other recipe you choose.

RECIPES FOR HEALTHY EYES

Chrysanthemum Flower Eye Wash   (yin)

Chrysanthemum flowers are valued for their antiseptic properties and are used to provide a cooling energy that not only eases inflammation and reduces swelling but also clears up eyes that are bloodshot from too much alcohol or smoke. You can also drink this golden liquid as a healing tea. Just add a bit of honey and enjoy.

Makes 3 treatments

   3 tablespoons dried chrysanthemum flowers (see NOTE)

Bring 3 cups of water to a boil. Add chrysanthemum flowers and stir to distribute them in the water. Reduce heat to medium and simmer until liquid is reduced to 2 cups.

   Cool to lukewarm. Pour 1 cup into a small bowl and pour the rest into a glass bottle or jar for future use. Stored in the refrigerator, this will keep for 1 week.

   Using either a small glass eyecup or cottonballs, soak your eyes for 2 to 3 minutes. Do not reuse eyewash.

NOTE: You can substitute honeysuckle flowers for this refreshing concoction. Both are available at herb shops and health food stores, or from the mail-order Resources listed on page 253.

Pearl Powder Milk   (yin)

Pearl powder may be exotic to you, but it is a special component of the beauty bag of tricks for most Asian women. Pearl powder really is made of ground-up pearls! This frothy drink helps nourish both the eyes and the skin. It is especially helpful for anyone who suffers from excessive mucus in the corners of their eyes. It's a lovely bedtime drink.

Makes 1 serving

    8 ounces hot milk
    ¼ teaspoon pearl powder (see NOTE)
    Honey to taste

Pour hot milk and pearl powder in a glass and mix well. Add honey to taste.

NOTE: Pearl powder is available at Asian markets and some health food stores, or from the mail-order Resources listed on page 253.

Bitter Melon and Beef in Black Bean Sauce   (yin/yang)

A popular Chinese dish, this intensely flavorful meal helps to cool excess heat energy in the body, especially in the liver. It uses a well-known detoxifying food, bitter melon, to stimulate the flow of chi to the liver. A delicious way to sharpen your eyesight, this dish is not recommended for people with digestion problems.

Makes 4 main-dish servings

1 medium bitter melon (see NOTE), cut in half lengthwise,
    seeds removed, and cut into ½-inch slices
2 tablespoons salt
3 tablespoons vegetable oil
3 to 4 cloves garlic, peeled and crushed
3 tablespoons fermented black beans (see NOTE)
2 tablespoons flour
1 pound lean beef (flank steak or top round sirloin), cut into 1-inch
    slices
2 tablespoons dry sherry
3 scallions, cut into 2-inch pieces
2 tablespoons soy sauce
1 tablespoon cornstarch

Bring 2 cups of water to a boil. Put melon slices in boiling water for 1 minute. Drain. Sprinkle with the salt and toss to coat slices with salt. Let sit for 15 minutes, then rinse in cold water to remove salt. Drain and set aside.

Heat 1 tablespoon oil in wok or large heavy skillet over high heat. Quickly stir-fry garlic and fermented black beans. Sprinkle flour over beef and toss to coat. Add 2 tablespoons oil to wok and quickly stir-fry meat for 3 to 5 minutes, until browned. Add sherry and continue cooking 1 minute. Add wax melon and scallions; stir to mix.

Stir in ¼ cup water and soy sauce. Reduce heat slightly and continue cooking.

Dissolve cornstarch in 2 tablespoons water and pour into beef-melon mixture. Stir until blended. When sauce has thickened, turn off heat and serve immediately.

Serve over rice, if desired.

NOTE: You can use 1 large regular cucumber, peeled, seeded, and cut into spears, if unable to buy bitter melon (available at Asian markets and some specialty grocery stores). Fermented black beans are available at Asian markets and health food stores.

Pork and Chinese Yam Congee   (yin/yang)

This wonderful dish helps brighten the eyes and strengthen the liver, spleen, and stomach. In fact, according to Chinese thinking, it helps nurture the body as a whole and stimulate the spirit. Chinese yams and wolfberries both promote kidney and liver function, making them two of the most commonly used ingredients in Chinese households.

Makes 4 main-dish servings

> 2 teaspoons dried wolfberries, soaked in warm water for 5 minutes
> 　　and drained
> ½ pound lean pork (pork loin or tenderloin), cut into 1-inch strips
> 2 medium pieces dried Chinese yam (see NOTE)
> ¾ cup rice
> 1-inch piece ginger, peeled and cut in half
> ½ cup chopped scallions
> 1 tablespoon soy sauce
> Salt and pepper to taste

Bring 6 cups of water, the wolfberries, pork, dried yam, rice, and ginger to a rolling boil in a 4-quart enamel soup pot. Reduce heat to medium and simmer for 25 minutes. Add the chopped scallions and stir. Add soy sauce and return to a boil for 5 minutes. Season with salt and pepper to taste.

NOTE: Dried Chinese yams, known as shanyao, are sold in herb shops and Asian markets by the piece. Unlike sweet potatoes and the more familiar golden yams, these tubers are white.

Chicken, Carrot, and Wolfberry Soup *(yin/yang)*

Wolfberries and carrots are probably the most important foods we can eat to improve our eyes. And we already know that chicken is not only tasty, it's a natural stomach healer. This is one of my family's all-time favorite soups. I'm sure you'll enjoy it, too.

Makes 4 to 6 main-dish servings

> One 2- to 3-pound chicken, or 4 whole chicken breasts
> 2 medium carrots, peeled and cut into ½-inch pieces
> 1 large onion, coarsely chopped
> 6 to 8 cloves garlic, peeled and crushed
> 1-inch piece ginger, peeled and cut in half
> 3 tablespoons dried wolfberries (see NOTE)
> 2 tablespoons soy sauce
> Salt and pepper to taste

Remove skin from chicken and cut into 1-inch pieces. Remove meat from bones if you prefer; however, chicken cooked with the bones is more nutritious.

Place chicken, carrots, onion, garlic, ginger, and wolfberries in a large enamel soup pot. Cover with 6 to 8 cups of water, making sure that all ingredients are submerged. Bring to a boil, reduce temperature to medium, and cover. Cook for 45 minutes to an hour, until chicken is tender. Add soy sauce, and salt and pepper to taste. Stir to combine.

NOTE: Dried wolfberries are available at Asian markets and health food stores, or from the mail-order Resources listed on page 253.

Pork Liver and Vegetable Soup   *(yin)*

The long list of ingredients belies the fact that this is a very easy soup to make. Not only is it exceptionally tasty but it is among the most nutritious soups you can make. The liver and garlic both work wonders for the eyes.

Makes 4 main-dish servings

> *Seasoning Mix*
> ½ teaspoon sugar
> 1 teaspoon sesame oil
> 1 tablespoon soy sauce
> 1 tablespoon cornstarch
>
> ½ pound lean pork loin, thinly sliced
> ½ pound pork liver, thinly sliced
> 3 teaspoons vegetable oil
> 2 cloves garlic, peeled and crushed
> 2-inch piece ginger, peeled and sliced
> 1 pound spinach, washed carefully and tough stems removed
> Salt to taste

Combine Seasoning Mix ingredients in a large bowl. Add pork and liver, and toss gently to cover. Cover bowl and set aside.

Heat a large, enamel soup pot, add the oil, and stir-fry the garlic and ginger for 2 minutes. Add 6 cups of water and bring to a boil. Add pork and liver; boil on high heat for 10 to 12 minutes, until meat is thoroughly cooked. Add spinach and continue cooking for an additional 5 minutes. Add salt to taste.

9.

MAKE UP WITH MAKEUP

COLOR AND CARE FOR YOUR PERFECT CANVAS

By now, you've probably gathered that *The Tao of Beauty* is not your traditional beauty book. Certainly I will share some of the secrets I've learned as a model and spa owner, but that's not the point. The point I want to make is that your beauty is already there within you; cosmetics are merely a way to enhance that beauty.

The Tao of beauty is not about amassing piles of products, but about finding the look that works best for you. It does not mean that the more cosmetics you own or use, the more beautiful you'll be. The best way is first to have beautiful, glowing skin. This, as we discussed in Chapter 5, is accomplished from the inside out by making sure that the entire body is in harmony. The systems of the body—especially the liver and kidneys—must be in vibrant good health for your natural beauty to be obvious.

While the traditional Chinese theory that health is beauty and vice versa is valid, it does not mean that we don't need a little assistance to perfect the picture.

I don't know of a woman, regardless of her culture, who did not play with her mother's makeup as a child. It must have something to do with our female genes. Even now, after my years as a model and beauty professional, I still love makeup for the way it can boost my morale, plus, let's face it, the self-assurance a little vanity brings.

Interestingly, though, my current cache of cosmetics is a mere fraction of what you'd expect a model or spa owner to own. I've whittled my bag of tricks down to a perfect core group of products that work for me. You can simplify your life by tossing out all your extraneous cosmetics, especially anything over a year old. If you have not used a makeup or skin-care product for a year, you aren't going to wake up one morning and start using it any time soon. Besides, the preservatives and stabilizers in most skin-care products and makeup are active for only so long after the product has been opened. Throw it out. Now.

WHAT'S RIGHT FOR YOU?

Once you find the basic makeup products that are right for you, you will begin to develop a beauty routine you can use now and for years to come. I suppose most of us have spent a lot of money buying makeup for the wrong reasons: it's fashionable, or it's a good deal, or most likely, the makeup salesperson recommended it. I'm going to show you how to buy makeup for the *right* reasons.

In my early modeling days, when I was in my late teens, I thought I could wear only certain colors. Well, my modeling experience proved me wrong! Makeup artists and fashion stylists have seen to it that I have worn every color in the rainbow. While there have been a few exceptions—very bright yellow and orange; some very pale shades of yellow, blue, and green; gray, especially close to my face—most have looked just fine. Of course, I must admit that some colors have looked much better than others.

The key to successfully selecting makeup colors is to identify the color group that best suits your skin tone and the color of your eyes and hair. The most important thing about cosmetics is to understand the two cosmetic color family groups: the cool or blue/pink family, the yin colors, and the warm, yellow/golden family, the yang colors. These two groups lie at opposite ends of the spectrum, with neutral in the middle. Think back to grade school, when you learned about the color wheel: yellow on one side, blue on the other, red in the middle.

Every color has its yin/cool and yang/warm aspect. For example, take red.

Red blended with a little blue—raspberry, mauve, pink, etc.—is on the yin or cool side. On the other hand, red blended with a little yellow—brick, coral, peach, etc.—is on the yang or warm side. Pure, primary red, with nothing added, in this case, we can call it neutral—in the middle. Before I confuse you completely, let me provide a color vocabulary:

- *Color* is the pigmentation or hue of an object. Red. Brown.
- *Shade* is the degree of darkness or lightness of this color. Light blue. Dark gray.
- *Tone* is the quality of this color. Green with a yellow undertone.

When we use these terms to describe makeup, color is relatively obvious—red, blue, green, black, etc. Shade and tone are a little less obvious. A shade of red might be dark or deep red, rose, or pink, while tone generally refers to other colors that play in the main color.

I have a friend who has very olive skin, and if she wears orange lipstick, the green undertone of her skin becomes pronounced, giving her skin a sickly cast.

Another friend has hair as dark red as an Irish setter's and porcelain, blue-toned skin. She has drawers filled with lipsticks, blushes, and shadows that make her look ill. She finally learned to stand her ground and insist on cool, yin colors that *complement* the blue cast to her skin instead of fighting it. Until then, makeup salesclerks pushed warm, yang peaches, oranges, and rusts—the colors most often associated with red hair—that looked harsh, even garish, against her blue-white skin. "This was a very expensive lesson," she confided. Of course, not all redheads are like her. I know of red-haired women with golden or peach undertones to their skin who look fantastic in rusts and oranges and browns.

I have a salon customer who, like my friend, has a lot of blue undertones in her creamy beige skin. Her biggest complaint is that almost every lipstick she tries turns purple or greenish brown. She now neutralizes this blueness by using an opaque foundation, feathering it to her hairline and lightly down her neck, then covering her lips to give a clean palette for her lip color. Now, when she applies her lipstick, the color stays true.

Remember: Cosmetic colors look different on everyone, particularly in lipsticks because of the pigmentation of the lips.

The following chart compares the cool and warm aspects of several common makeup colors. Initially you may see similarities, but give them some thought. A pale pink and delicate peach, or turquoise and jade, at first glance, may appear the same; however, the pink and turquoise have distinctly cool properties, and the peach and jade, decidedly warm tones.

COOL AND WARM MAKEUP COLORS

COOL (YIN) COLORS	WARM (YANG) COLORS
Cherry Red	Brick Red
Purple	Magenta
Pink	Peach
Baby Blue	Aqua
Turquoise	Jade
Lemon Yellow	Banana
Forest Green/Dark Spruce Green	Grass/Lime
White	Ivory
Gray	Beige

Skin colors and undertones can also be studied in the context of coolness, warmth, and balance. The next chart compares skin tones with a spectrum of cosmetic colors.

SKIN TONE AND COSMETIC COLOR SPECTRUMS

YIN/COOL	BALANCED	YANG/WARM
Skin Colors		
White	Neutral/Tan	Peach
Purple/Black	Medium Brown	Golden Brown
Undertones		
Blue	Neutral	Peach
Green	Neutral	Yellow
Makeup Colors		

Blue → Purple → Magenta → Pink → **Red** ← Brown ← Brick ← Orange ← Yellow

DEVELOP YOUR OWN MAKEUP ROUTINE

The first step in establishing your makeup regimen is to determine the basic color family that is most appropriate to your beauty profile. I will not use a season of the year, an obscure color palette, or any other complicated, gimmicky system; I prefer to keep things simple.

Through the years, I'm sure that I've undergone more odd color analyses than any other woman on this planet. This is precisely why, when formulating my own color and cosmetics line for my spa, I wanted to avoid complicated or arbitrary classification systems myself. So get ready for the clearest, most concise color cosmetics profile ever!

As the charts on page 173 show, every color—like everything else—has a yin and a yang aspect, the opposite ends of the same spectrum. Yin colors are cool blue tones derived from the midnight blue color around the moon. Yang colors are derived from the yellow of the sun. This beautiful, and I think quite lyrical, natural color dichotomy is met in the middle by a whole family of neutral shades, including white, taupe, beige, and other pale tones.

DETERMINE YOUR COLORS

How can you determine whether your essential color family is yin or yang? The surest way is to analyze your skin tone and the color of your eyes or hair. Is the main undertone of your skin pink or blue? If so, you're a cool yin. On the other hand, if your skin is yellow or olive, you're most probably a warm yang.

If you are still not sure which color family will look most natural on you, comb your hair back and study your face in a well-lit mirror. Drape a white towel across your chest so that there will be no reflected color to influence what you are seeing. Take a close look at the *colors* in your eyes. (Note the plural.) Splashed through every eye color—blue, brown, hazel, even lilac—are dazzling flecks of gold, silver, and copper, as well as blue, brown, red, yellow, and even green. This gives you an incredible selection of colors to choose from that will *enhance* your features rather than detract from their beauty.

One salon client claimed that she never used eye shadows and liners because they always made her blue eyes look dull and gray. When I asked her what colors she had used, she said blue-gray and slate blue. No wonder. She was using two trendy shades of the same color, both very close to the intense blue of her eyes, resulting in a faded, lifeless look. When I introduced her to a golden rose shadow that picked up the rich gold sparkle I saw in her eyes and gave her a warm mahogany liner and mascara, her eyes popped to life. They were dazzling. The blue and gray tones she had used previously were too close to the primary blue color of her eyes, while the golden tones I recommended brought out the rich undertones that enhanced the regal blue of her eyes.

Another way to figure out your color family is to take a look at your closet. It says a lot about you. We naturally gravitate to the colors that make us feel good, that we know help make us *look* good, so you probably have a core wardrobe of flattering colors. Considering only the clothes that you wear, the colors that make you look beautifully alive, ask: Do I wear more cool or warm shades? Is my wardrobe full of navy, sapphire, purple—cool, yin colors? Or are there more clothes in the browns, tans, oranges, and reds—warm, yang colors?

If you still can't decide if your color family is yin or yang by looking in the mirror or at your wardrobe, get two blouses or two pieces of fabric large enough to drape around your neck in front. One should be pure white, the other ivory. Hold them up to your face, one at a time. If you feel better and look more beautiful in one than the other, you will know which color family is best suited for you. Notice how clear white has a blue, cool, tone and the ivory/beige has a yellow, warm, tone.

If you're like me, you may be happy with either color group, depending on your disposition or your physical condition. But be cautious with your color choices. Take care not to select extreme colors at either end of the spectrum. Cosmetic choices really depend on an individual's lifestyle, feelings, and level of comfort. If you work in a restaurant at night or are in a creative field, you might feel best wearing stronger, more theatrical colors, whereas if you work days in a bookstore or a conservative office you might feel more comfortable wearing softer, more natural, neutral colors.

While I feel that most women can wear colors from either family, it is definitely best to wear all cool, or all warm, at the same time. For example, if you use a bright coral lipstick, which is warm in its color energy, with a rosy blush, and then apply ruby and gray shadows, two cool yin hues, the result is rather clownish, especially if you've used a creamy beige foundation.

If you are not feeling your best, your skin's undertones may be more visible than when your body is in balance and in good health. One client came to my spa for a makeover not long after having knee surgery. Mary complained that she was tired of looking "drab." Indeed, her skin was dull and lifeless, with a greenish yellow cast to it. We discussed her overall health, including the medications she was taking. I explained to her that once she was healthy, her skin color would probably change, so we'd want to take that into consideration when selecting her makeup color scheme. I suggested that she wait until she was off the medications before making any decision about changing her hair color—which she had wanted to do—and makeup palette. About six weeks later, Mary came into the spa with a smile on her face. "You were right," she said. "I don't look like I'm turning into a green space alien any more."

As Mary's body healed and was restored to balance, the blue undertones in her fair skin were no longer overshadowed by the jaundiced yellow cast caused by imbalances in her liver. Knowing that she had a yin complexion made it possible for me to create a makeup palette that suited Mary's coloring and gave her a variety of beautiful makeup looks.

MAKEUP COLORS

Lipstick colors in the cool (yin) family have names such as pink, rose, mauve, plum, ruby, sherry, roseberry, raspberry, wine, and magenta. Lipsticks in the warm (yang) family have names like brandy, peach, coral, crimson, mocha, persimmon, russet, cognac, toffee, cappuccino, terra cotta, brick, nectarine, or ginger.

Look at the shade of your favorite foundation, the one that makes your skin look its loveliest. This is a very good way to learn if your best color family is yin or yang. Many companies label their products with names that include the notation "cool" or "warm." In this case, your work's a snap because you'll know beyond a shadow of a doubt if you're using a yin or yang foundation. When a foundation color is right, it blends easily, so that there is no dramatic line of demarcation between your face, hairline, and neck. Your skin color will complement your hair color, and your eyes will look clear, providing a beautifully natural-looking palette.

Even lacking this specific information, the name of your foundation color still provides clues. Does it have peach or bronze on the label? Chances are, it's a yang. Conversely, if it has rose or pink on the label, it's yin.

But don't stop there. Make sure you're choosing the right cool or warm colors by considering these next points.

With a few exceptions, almost anyone can wear any color. It's a question of wearing those shades within that general color quality that look best on you. For instance, when it comes to red, a cool (yin) woman looks best in raspberry or watermelon shades—reds with blue tones. A warm (yang) woman looks best in an orange or brick-red shade, one with a yang tone.

MORE ABOUT SKIN TONES

Need more proof that skin tone, not hair color, should determine your cosmetics palette? Then consider these famous blondes: Cybill Shepherd is a classic yellow-skinned, golden blonde who looks fabulous in shades of apricot, chartreuse, and sunshine yellow; her everyday makeup should thus be in the warm family. Candice Bergen, on the other hand, is also a Scandinavian blonde, but one with a cool cast to her skin. She looks softer and prettier in mid-range blues and greens. Warm makeup colors would appear jarring on her skin, whereas pink and rosy blushers bring out the natural color in her cheeks.

All that said, there's an interesting point-counterpoint dimension to my views on color:

- When you want to achieve a soft, naturally becoming look, use colors from your own group.
- When you want to create a dramatic glamour look, you have two choices—more intense shades from your specific color group, or shades from the opposite color group.
- Again, take care to stay within the same color family: Yin foundation with yin blush, eye colors, and mascara; yang with yang. As I've said, mixing the two is garish rather than glamorous.

Whether you choose the natural or dramatic look, keep the tonalities constant for the most beautiful and appealing results.

No matter what colors you choose, always aim for a clean, clear look. Remember those disco war-paint "cheekbones" from the 1970s? Thankfully, they and other heavy-handed sculpting and contouring techniques are things of the past.

Today's makeup is about enhancing and highlighting your best points. It's about bringing out a look of health, rather than seeking to change the shape of your face. Shading and contouring can work in some instances—in front of a television camera or for high-fashion photography. However, I certainly suggest avoiding such a dramatic look for daytime, as do many of the best-known makeup artists. They use palettes not of avant-garde, seasonal colors, but of basic neutrals that bring out the best in a woman's face. Did you know that 80 percent of the fashion shades introduced each year by cosmetics houses never become part of their ongoing lines? They may fit into a seasonal color scheme based on European fashions but are virtually unwearable in our everyday lives. In fact, the lion's share of makeup shades I wore on runways and in photo shoots during my modeling career was downright circuslike. I'd never wear those colors in real life. Remember this always: Out on the catwalk is not the same as out on the street! A fashion show is a show, not real life.

ASK FOR HELP IF YOU NEED IT

If you still need a little professional assistance with makeup colors, by all means get it—for free! Every department store cosmetics counter offers free makeovers, sometimes calling in national experts for in-store appearances. Spend an afternoon with a girlfriend (preferably one who's opinionated and not afraid to provide an honest point of view) and make the rounds of makeup counters. Unless specified otherwise, you can enjoy a makeover at absolutely no charge and with no purchase required.

Sometimes a professional makeup artist will uncover a whole new you by looking at your face in a totally objective light . . . but watch your wallet. Let the makeup artist know that, for now, you plan to buy only one or two new products—the most fundamental to your makeover—to experiment with at home. This establishes, right up front, that you will not be pressured into buying more makeup than you want, need, or will use.

YOUR BASIC BEAUTY NEEDS

Many of my spa clients have asked me for a basic makeup purchase plan. This is a pleasure, since I've always believed in simplicity. With makeup, less can be more. After years of modeling and formulating my own makeup line, I believe the following elements are all that a woman needs to present a beautiful, luminous face to the world:

1. **A makeup bag.** Since we use a makeup bag every day, buy one that is not only pretty but durable. This is one item that's worth spending a bit of money on, because the good ones last longer and are much nicer to use. It can make you feel inspired to open it and make yourself look beautiful. While I have seen many lovely, light-colored cosmetics carriers, I advise against them. Inevitably, they get dirty too quickly. Stick to colored bags—prints, patterns, navy, and classic black.

2. **An excellent foundation.** Foundation should match your skin tone as closely as possible; attempting to correct or change your skin tone can result in a major mistake. Your goal should always be to mimic your natural skin perfectly. It is much easier to buy this product in department stores and high-end pharmacies, because you can actually try on the products. The most important step is to check out your foundation in natural light. Make no exceptions to this rule, especially since the fancier the store, the more subdued the lighting! A quick dash outside ensures that the foundation will end up on your face and not stashed in the bottom drawer of your vanity. Also note that if you tend to tan in the summer, you will need a slightly darker shade of your regular foundation for that time of year.

You might also take advantage of one of my favorite new services: custom-blended cosmetics. For only slightly more money than the high-end cosmetics lines, you can have a foundation mixed to your exact skin tone. I've seen this service in better department stores, cosmetic chain stores, and even larger neighborhood drugstores.

3. **Eye shadows.** This is where many women tend to overpurchase or use only one shade out of an eye-shadow quartet. Such a waste! Drugstore and department store lines both offer a wide range of single- and double-pan shadows.

Generally speaking, two or three colors are all any woman needs. These should include one neutral tone (beige for deep-set eyes, taupe or brown for prominent eyes) and as a highlighter for under the brows. If you wish to add complementary tones to the brow bone (crease), you may add another color. Always be sure the colors remain in your basic yin or yang range.

I suggest that blue-toned yin women stick to pinks, reds, and blues, while yellow-hued yangs opt for corals, browns, and greens. In either case, always choose the most natural, neutral shades. Use fashion colors and glitter shadows for accents or glamorous functions only.

Here again, note that some colors have cousins in both the cool and warm ranges, with green as the perfect example. Cool-skinned yin women with blue, green, or hazel eyes may well want to try cool aqua or green shadows, whereas warm-skinned yang women look terrific in khaki green.

4. **Blush.** Two are all you need. Blush should provide a healthy, natural glow. With blush, less is always more. It should not appear on your cheeks like experimental modern art! Consider it an enhancement to your looks, not something that has a personality all its own.

I recommend using blush tones that complement your lipstick colors. If you're like me and wear makeup colors from both color families, don't confuse them and wear cheek color from one family and lipstick or eyeshadows from the other. Match lipstick and blush tones.

5. **Lipstick.** Here's where I get really revolutionary: All you need are two lipsticks plus one tube of pearly metallic—silver or gold. Let's face it,

most of us wear only one or two colors. Why have six or seven or more? One should be a natural shade in your yin or yang palette. The other should be a deeper, nighttime hue. I can already see you shaking your heads: How can a former model live with just two lipsticks? Easy. I can change the color by blending the two tubes with my lip brush. Besides, this makes me use them up before I rush out and buy new shades, which of course I love to do.

As for the special pearlized silver or gold lipstick: I sometimes blend it in the center of my lips to make them look shinier and fuller. I also mix it with my other lipsticks for a dramatic change.

6. **Face powder.** Use loose powder at home—it goes on smoother and is wonderfully luxurious—and keep a pressed powder in your purse for touch-ups during the day. I recommend buying top-quality powders from a makeup salon or department store, not because they're better than drugstore products, but because they come in a wider variety of shades. The very best way to select loose powder is to have it custom blended. This service is becoming more and more available, so it's worth a few phone calls to find a store that can do this.

Many cosmetics lines now have powders that match foundations. Rather than buying the traditional dark, medium, or light shade, you can buy a powder that's "light-cool" or "medium-warm," so you stay well within the confines of your skin type.

7. **Mascara.** Never keep a tube of mascara longer than six months. Even if you cap it tightly and wash the wand after use, it is likely to become a breeding ground for bacteria and other germs. The good news is this: Since no woman needs more than one mascara and this is a product most of us use every day, a tube shouldn't last more than three or four months anyway. Black is the most popular—and most practical—color. A neutral tone does the job.

You can also purchase mascara in brown-black, dark brown, brown, light brown, navy, clear, even in a rainbow of fashion or novelty colors. It's your choice.

Use mascara lightly for daytime and add an extra coat for dress-up occasions.

8. **Pencils.** All you need are four: one for your brows, one for your eyes, and one or two lip-liners. Because these products are basics, they should stay within your basic yin or yang color range. Resist the temptation to stray outside your basic color family.

    Here's a great inside tip: Virtually all lip, brow, and eyeliner pencils are made in one of a half dozen German factories; thus, there is absolutely no reason to go crazy searching for the brand that has the "best" pencil. My only recommendation is that you avoid some of the low-priced brands found in low-end drug- or discount stores. They might cake, or break when you sharpen them. Some can be too dry, which can hurt your eyes, or so greasy that they run into your eyes.

9. **Cosmetics pencil sharpener.** Here's where a bit of luck is needed. Sometimes an inexpensive pencil sharpener—the kind with both large and small openings—works great. But try several before buying one; you don't want a sharpener that will eat up your wonderful pencil. It is important to get a sharp sharpener for a strong point so that you don't ruin your pencil. There's no hard and fast rule. Regardless of where you buy the sharpener, use it often. A sharp pencil is much easier to control and is much more sanitary than a dull, overused pencil.

10. **Makeup brushes and other tools.** This is another area where I urge you to splurge. Free giveaways, cheap drugstore brushes, and almost all brushes that comes prepackaged with blushers or shadows are best avoided. You don't have to be a professional to see greatly improved results when you opt for high-quality makeup tools.

    This is one case where the adage "A good carpenter never blames his tools" is way off base! Where makeup brushes are concerned, the better the brush, the better the results.

    You'll need five good pony-hair or sable brushes in a variety of sizes to apply smooth, professional-quality makeup.

    - A small, firm, angled brush to line your eyes and shape your brows.
    - A medium-size flat brush for eye-shadow application. Use the side edge for detail and the flat side to apply shadow. This one is good for blending.

- A small flat brush for eye shadow. Use for more control and detail work.
- A medium-size blusher brush.
- A large, fluffy brush for powder.

A good brush deserves to be treated with respect, so be sure to wash your brushes often. I recommend using a gentle liquid soap in warm water to dissolve skin and makeup oils. Add a little bit of hair conditioner to the rinse water. Press the water out of the brushes and use your fingers to gently mold them back into their original shapes.

A MODEL'S MAKEUP TIPS

- Use a creamy concealer or an eye makeup base before applying shadow. This will ensure that the makeup lasts longer.
- Use foundation and concealer sparingly, or lines and creases will become more pronounced.
- Choose concealer that is the same color—or lighter—than your foundation. Just make sure that it is in the same color family as your skin.
- Use loose powder sparingly, as it can be drying, and if you've overused foundation, it will make lines and creases more obvious.
- Avoid sparkling or pearly eye-makeup colors. They tend to make your eyes look puffy.
- Take care when applying liner under your eyes. Heavy dark lines tend to make you look hard or mean rather than beautiful and seductive.
- Open your eyes by brushing a light neutral shadow on the outside of your upper eyelids, up under the brows.
- Stay away from greens, blues, or any other deep eye shadow colors that require great skill to blend. Shadows should enhance your eyes, not call attention to themselves.
- For a fresh, natural look, select shadow and blush colors that are close to your skin color and tone, only deeper or lighter, depending on how you'll be using them.

- Select colors that warm or brighten your skin tone—golden tan or rosy pink blush tones, for example. Always apply makeup in upward, outward strokes for an uplifting, happier effect. Downward strokes make you look tired and unhappy.
- Smile, then brush blusher onto the "apples" of your cheeks in feathery upward, outward strokes.
- For an "instant facelift," apply a lighter tone of foundation under your eyes and over the "laugh lines" below your nose and around your mouth. Then blend regular foundation to create a clear, smooth face. Use a light touch of liner close to your upper lashes to give the illusion of thick lashes, and then apply mascara to your upper lashes. Holding your mascara wand vertically, apply just a touch to your lower lashes (remove the excess or clumps from your lashes with a lash comb or cotton swab).
- Make your lips appear fuller and more sensual by brushing a light coat of silver (yin) or gold (yang) lipstick on the center of your bottom lip.

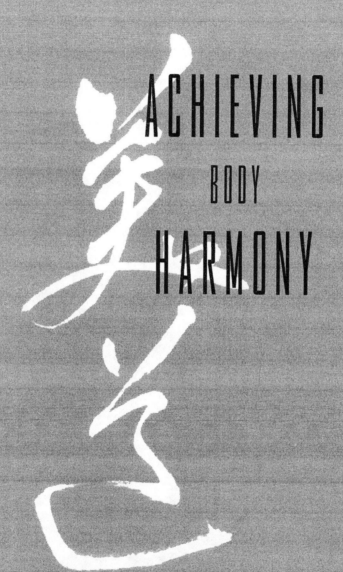

ACHIEVING
BODY
HARMONY

10.

EXERCISES FOR ENERGY

CHI KUNG KEEPS YOU
YOUTHFUL, HEALTHY, AND BEAUTIFUL

Exercise is a vital component of any beauty routine, regardless of its origin, and it's absolutely essential to a Chinese beauty-wellness program. While I don't insist that my spa clients do all the same exercises I do, I highly recommend a powerful set of breathing exercises and connected movements from an ancient Chinese practice known as *Chi Kung.*

A 3000-year-old Chinese healing exercise discipline, *Chi Kung* is practiced in various forms by people of all ages. You may have seen it performed on *National Geographic* TV specials about China—elderly women and men gracefully moving in flowing, precise sweeps. It is as much a part of Chinese culture as the theory of yin and yang, and it is a growing part of Western culture as well.

Chi means energy or internal energy, and is sometimes translated as breath. The word *Kung* means work, practice, or exercise. *Chi Kung*—energy exercise— combines slow, precise movements, powerful, controlled deep breathing, and sounds that increase the flow of blood and *chi* to the vital organs. This removes any energy blockages that may be causing stagnation of the blood and *chi. Chi*

Kung exercises are designed to cultivate a strong life energy system by rebalancing and strengthening *chi*.

Chi Kung was developed thousands of years ago as a ritual healing dance by early Taoist monks, who perfected breathing methods and flowing postures to purify and preserve the body. An early Confucian writing, *Spring and Autumn Annals,* states, "Flowing water never stagnates. The hinges of an active door never rust. This is due to movement. The same principle applies to essence and energy. If the body does not move, *chi* does not flow, and energy stagnates." This is the principle behind *Chi Kung.*

Hundreds of *Chi Kung* disciplines have been handed down through the centuries, both by oral tradition and in ancient writings. One of the earliest of these, the "Play of the Five Animals," is based on observations of animals and their movements—shoulder postures are inspired by the movement of bears; arm exercises reflect the way birds flap their wings; leg exercises emulate a tiger's pounce, and so on. Most exercises, regardless of the discipline, begin with the "Stance of the Horse." Stand straight with your weight evenly distributed and feet slightly apart. Knees should be relaxed and slightly bent, and arms should hang loosely at your sides. Other postures capture the movements of the dragon, snake, and phoenix.

Chi Kung has four basic benefits: health and well-being, long life, martial power, and spiritual enlightenment. And, as with many Taoist exercises, there are many paths to accomplish each. For simplicity's sake, we will deal only with exercises that promote beauty and longevity. The exercises I share in this chapter are a mere sampling of the many powerful *Chi Kung* movements that exercise the body inside and out.

EAST MEETS WEST TO EXERCISE

The Chinese take a very yin, or passive, approach to exercise. To them, exercise is for revitalizing the body as the Organic Whole. In the West, exercise emphasizes competitiveness and exertion. Even supposedly solitary sports, like running, stress the body to its utmost limits, a very yang practice. Such sudden and dramatic physical stress often results in injury.

I shudder when I hear someone say, "No pain, no gain" or "Go for the burn." How dangerous and even counterproductive these adages are. I caution my spa clients to view their bodies not as an opponent to be conquered, but rather as a friend to be cultivated. I have witnessed how they ignore signals like burning and cramping; signals that are telling them to slow down. Instead of listening, many of my clients push their bodies to go beyond what is comfortable or even productive. They ignore their body's pleas; then, with overtaxed muscles and stressed joints, they injure themselves severely. Sometimes permanently.

I understand the American quest for the perfect body. When I was modeling full-time, I was keenly aware of how many people in the beauty business thought that one was never thin enough, pretty enough, or young enough. I too gave in to this absurd, even dangerous, pressure to be physically "perfect" and followed the lead of some of the models I worked with. At nineteen years old, I started jogging, rain or shine. I was adamant about getting in my daily three miles, even when I was traveling. If I couldn't get to a track, beach, or running trail, I jogged up and down the airport lobby or hotel corridors. It took shin-splints so painful that I was in danger of losing the job I loved—modeling on the fashion runways—for me to take a second look at running as my primary form of exercise. I was in such excruciating pain that I couldn't wear high heels and had difficulty walking properly. It was only then that I realized I couldn't force myself to be the runner I was not. So I returned to the ancient *Chi Kung* exercises that my grandmother and mother taught me.

I cannot promise that *Chi Kung* will give you eternal youth, wealth, and prosperity, as the ancients claimed it could, but I can assure you that if you listen to your body and respect its needs and limits, exercising it gently and faithfully every day, optimum health and beauty will be yours.

CHI KUNG FOR BUSY WOMEN

The following *Chi Kung* exercises have been adapted to fit the busy schedules of today's working mothers and professionals, and anyone else who wants to preserve youth, increase stamina, and build *chi* to its fullest potential. These movements are simple, easy to do, and once you have mastered them, they should take no more than thirty minutes a day.

The Chinese take the practice of *Chi Kung* very seriously, more seriously than any other form of exercise. It is an exercise of the *chi,* the energy and spirit, and like any creative discipline, must be done consciously and correctly. It is not to be approached lightly.

This *Chi Kung* program has been broken down into five basic routines to be perfected over a period of five weeks. You will spend the first week practicing the most basic exercise, which concentrates on increasing *chi* in the lungs. Week Two builds on this basic lung exercise and adds an exercise for the liver, and Week Three expands the program to include an exercise for the kidneys. During Week Four, you will combine the three previous exercises with one that affects the heart, and during Week Five you will add an exercise for the spleen. By the sixth week, *Chi Kung* should be a solid part of your beauty-wellness program and you'll be feeling its wonderful effects.

I also offer *Chi Kung* exercises for your face—something you can do anytime, anyplace, when you need a pick-me-up—and a quick relaxing sequence that is guaranteed to remove tension from your head and neck so that you can relax and get a good night's sleep.

For the following *Chi Kung* exercises, you can sit or stand, depending on your health and physical condition. If you need to do these exercises sitting down, do so. As you build strength, you will become strong enough to perform them standing. After all, the purpose of *Chi Kung* is to increase your energy and stamina, not wear you out.

GROUND RULES BEFORE EXERCISING

Here are some important things to remember when embarking on your exercise program:

1. Do not exercise when you are not feeling well, even with a minor cold. Because *Chi Kung* stimulates the flow of *chi* throughout the body, it can cause stress that could delay recuperation.

2. Do *Chi Kung* once a day, preferably in the morning. Without the stresses of the day to occupy your thoughts, you will be more relaxed, and with your mind clear and calm, you'll be more able to control your breathing.

3. Do not exercise during your menstrual cycle. These exercises might cause an extremely heavy flow.

4. Do not exercise on an empty stomach, or on a full stomach either. Wait about two hours after a big meal and an hour after a light meal before beginning an exercise session.

5. For best results, eat foods that provide the best possible fuel for this intense form of exercise—fresh fruits and vegetables, whole grains. Avoid fried foods, dairy products, and overeating in general.

6. Before exercising, empty your bladder. Do not urinate immediately after *Chi Kung,* even if you feel the need. Try to wait five minutes to allow the energy generated during your exercise session to be absorbed by your body.

7. Before exercising, remove all jewelry and loosen belts and constricting clothes. Anything that presses against the body can inhibit the powerful *Chi Kung* breathing and obstruct energy flow.

8. Always wear comfortable clothes and soft, flexible shoes. Again, this allows for full movement of your body.

9. Do not practice *Chi Kung* after doing other types of strenuous exercise. Your body needs to be calm and rested to benefit from this program.

10. Avoid doing *Chi Kung* close to bedtime. If you do practice close to bedtime, your body may not be receptive to sleep.

11. Do not breathe heated or air-conditioned air directly while doing *Chi Kung.* Such extreme temperatures can be excessively drying to the lungs.

12. Some fresh air is ideal while practicing *Chi Kung,* but don't overdo it. *Chi Kung* opens your energy meridians so thoroughly that if you exercise in a windy area, you can open your body to wind/chill problems such as bloating, joint pain, and heavy-headedness.

13. Keep your spirit calm and peaceful while doing *Chi Kung.* If you are emotionally upset, you will scatter energy, which is potentially harmful when practicing *Chi Kung.*

14. Focus on your breathing while doing *Chi Kung*. This, in turn, will calm your spirit, open your heart, and relax your body and mind.

15. Never shower or bathe immediately after a *Chi Kung* exercise session. Done correctly, these movements will open your pores and make you perspire. Wait at least a half hour to give your pores time to close, and give the *chi* that will be circulating vigorously through your body time to be absorbed. To shower or bathe too soon after exercising opens you to attacks of dampness and cold energy—from cramping, bloating, and joint pain to fuzzy thinking, vaginal discharge, and cold hands and feet. In Chinese practice, bathing or showering immediately after a body massage is not recommended for similar reasons. My baby sister learned this lesson the hard way. When she started doing *Chi Kung* exercises, she was already accustomed to regular exercise. She took aerobic classes at the gym and was a runner—two very yang, or active, exercise programs. One day after a *Chi Kung* session, she changed out of her exercise clothes and hopped into the shower, just as she would after an aerobic workout. As a result, she had chills for two full days. It took a lot of ginger tea to restore warmth to her body.

THE BASIC CHI KUNG PROGRAM

As I have said, *Chi Kung* takes discipline and concentration. Set aside time every day for the next five weeks—in the morning, if at all possible—to learn these powerful, energizing moves.

Spend the first week doing the basic *chi* or balanced *chi* exercise; then add one exercise a week for the next four weeks until you are doing all five exercises in combination.

If you are unable to do any part of these exercises while standing, sit on the side of your bed or on a sturdy, straight-back chair. As you begin the practice of *Chi Kung,* you may find that you tire quickly. Should that happen, take a break and, once you're rested, resume exercising.

TUNING INTO THE POWER OF THE BREATH

Do you ever pay attention to how you breathe? In my experience, most people don't, unless they have asthma or some other respiratory condition. It's almost as if they've forgotten how to listen to the breath.

Breathing is an essential component of *Chi Kung*. The following exercises will teach you to breathe deeply and calmly to draw energy into the body. You will learn to use your diaphragm and abdominal muscles as pumps, drawing breath way down into your lungs. Such deep breathing pulls energy through the meridians, or energy centers, to totally empower your body with *chi*. Inhale through your nose, using your diaphragm to pull air deeply into your lungs, then expel the breath through your mouth, vocalizing the sound assigned to each exercise. You'll be using your abdominal muscles to push the air from your body.

Keep a box of tissues handy when doing your *Chi Kung* exercises. You'll probably need them—especially if you're a beginner—to clear your nasal passages as you strengthen your breath. *Chi Kung* is also helpful for snorers. Keep a tall glass or bottle of cool or warm (never cold) water at hand to sip while exercising. Drink as much and as often as you need during the breaks between sets to maintain the flow of fluids through your body.

FIRST WEEK

This is the basic chi *or balanced* chi *exercise.*

Target: The lungs
Breathing: Take strong, deep breaths in and out through your nose.

Steps:
1. Stand straight. Find your center, standing with your feet slightly apart, knees relaxed and slightly bent.

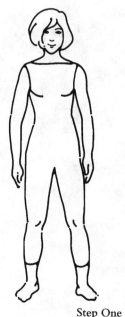

Step One

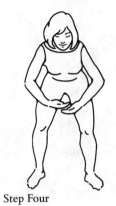

Step Four

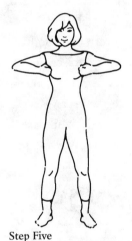

Step Five

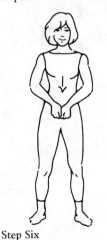

Step Six

2. Let your shoulders relax and your arms hang loosely at your sides.

3. Stretch your arms out to the side at shoulder level. Relax your hands. Turn your thumbs up and your palms forward to expand your chest and open your lungs.

4. Inhale deeply through your nose as you bend forward from the waist and, reaching toward the floor, scoop up an armful of energy, hugging it to your body with your hands, as you return to a standing position, straightening your spine until you are standing upright. As you gather energy, curl your fingers into your palms to form fists.

5. Extend your elbows out to the sides and turn your fists so that they are facing each other at chest level.

6. Bring your fists together against your chest, then turn them downward and press the *chi* down into your torso while forcing air through your nostrils.

7. Return to starting position.

Repetitions: Do 6 sets of 6 repetitions every day for the first week. Sip water between sets if desired. Once you have mastered the exercise, it should take about 15 minutes to complete this routine.

SECOND WEEK

Do this exercise in sequence with the basic chi *exercise learned during the first week.*

Target: The liver
Breathing: Inhale deeply through the nose and force

the air from your lungs as you make the sound *shhhh* to balance the *chi* as it exits your liver.

Steps:

1. Stand straight. Find your center, standing with your feet slightly apart, knees relaxed and slightly bent.
2. Let your shoulders relax and your arms hang loosely at your sides.
3. Stretch your arms out to the side at shoulder level. Relax your hands. Turn your thumbs up and your palms forward to expand your chest and open your lungs.
4. Inhale deeply through your nose as you bend forward from the waist and, reaching toward the floor, scoop up an armful of energy, hugging it to your body with your hands, as you return to a standing position. As you gather energy, curl your fingers into your palms to form fists.
5. Extend your elbows out to the side and turn your fists toward each other at chest level.
6. Rather than pressing *chi* downward, turn your fists upward, over your head; your elbows should be parallel, about four to eight inches apart.
7. Slowly curl your body forward, dropping your head as you slowly exhale through your mouth making a *shhhh* sound.
8. Slowly uncurl upward into starting position.

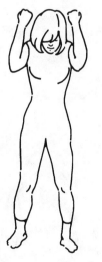

Step Seven

Repetitions: Do 3 exercises for the lungs followed by 3 exercises for the liver; rest for 30 seconds and repeat this sequence 6 times. This session should take about 20 minutes. Always end with another exercise for the lungs to balance *chi*.

THIRD WEEK

This is done in sequence with the exercises learned in the first two weeks.

Target: The kidneys

Breathing: Inhale through your nose as you begin this exercise. As you exhale, force air from your lungs with the sound *phoo,* like you are blowing out a candle. This sound is known to release tension and balance *chi* in the kidneys.

Steps:

1. Stand straight. Find your center, standing with your feet slightly apart, knees relaxed and slightly bent.
2. Let your shoulders relax and your arms hang loosely at your sides.
3. Stretch your arms out to the side at shoulder level. Relax your hands. Turn your thumbs up and your palms forward to expand your chest and open your lungs.
4. Inhale deeply through your nose as you bend forward from the waist and, reaching toward the floor, scoop up an armful of energy, hugging it to your body with your hands as you return to a standing position. As you gather energy, curl your fingers into your palms to form fists.

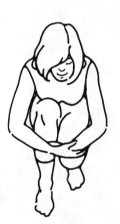

Step Eight

5. Extend your elbows out to the side and turn your fists toward each other at chest level.
6. Inhale deeply through your nose as you step forward with your right leg.
7. Bend your right knee and slowly kneel down as far as you can.
8. Slowly curl your shoulders forward and tuck your chin in as you gently hug your right knee.
9. Exhale, using your abdominal muscles to slowly expel air from your body with a vigorous *phoo* sound through your mouth.
10. Slowly return to starting position.

11. Do one lung, or basic *chi,* exercise, then repeat the above steps with your left leg forward.

Repetitions: Do 3 lung, or basic *chi,* exercises followed by 3 exercises for the liver, then 3 exercises for the kidneys. Rest for 30 seconds and repeat this sequence 6 times. This session should take about 20 minutes. End with an additional basic *chi* exercise.

FOURTH WEEK

This is done in sequence with the exercises mastered during the preceding three weeks.

Target: The heart
Breathing: Inhale through your nose as you begin this part of the exercise. As you exhale, force air from your lungs with the sound, *ha.* This sound balances *chi* in the heart and dispels excess heat.

Steps:
1. Stand straight. Find your center, standing with your feet slightly apart, knees relaxed and slightly bent.
2. Let your shoulders relax and your arms hang loosely at your sides.
3. Stretch your arms out to the side at shoulder level. Relax your hands. Turn your thumbs up and your palms forward to expand your chest and open your lungs.
4. Inhale deeply through your nose as you bend forward from the waist and, reaching toward the floor, scoop up an armful of energy, hugging it to your body with your hands.
5. Slowly return to a standing position and raise your arms upward. Open your hands, palms forward, as you stretch your arms over your head.
6. Look upward and lift your body up on the balls of your feet.

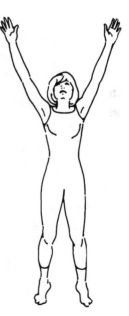

Step Six

7. Expel air through your mouth with a strong *ha* sound.
8. Slowly lower your arms and return to starting position.

Repetitions: Do 3 lung, or basic *chi,* exercises followed by 3 exercises for the liver, then 3 exercises for the kidneys and 3 exercises for the heart. Rest for 30 seconds and repeat this sequence 6 times. End with an additional basic *chi* exercise. This entire session should take about 20 minutes.

FIFTH WEEK

This exercise is done in sequence with all the previously learned exercises.

Target: The spleen

Breathing: Inhale through your nose as you begin this part of the exercise. As you exhale, force air from your lungs through your nostrils in quick, short breaths corresponding with the side you are exercising. This technique balances the *chi* in the spleen.

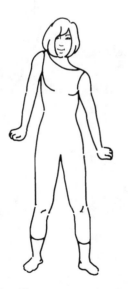

Step Five

Steps:
1. Stand straight. Find your center, standing with your feet slightly apart, knees relaxed and slightly bent.
2. Let your shoulders relax and your arms hang loosely at your sides.
3. Move arms up not quite halfway to shoulder level. Raise hands and wrists to shoulder level with the elbows slightly bent. Think of a partially opened umbrella.
4. Turn your palms forward and close your fingers into fists. Now turn the fists backward.
5. Take a strong inhale through your nose as you push your left shoulder downward so that you stretch to your right side. Then strongly exhale

as you press your right arm downward to stretch your left side. Do 10 stretches. Slowly return to starting position.

6. Do one lung, or basic *chi,* exercise. Then repeat this exercise, starting by stretching to the right.

Repetitions: Do 3 lung, or basic *chi,* exercises followed by 3 exercises for the liver; then 3 exercises for the lungs, 3 exercises for the kidneys, 3 exercises for the lungs, 3 exercises for the heart, and 3 exercises for the lungs, 3 exercises for the spleen. Rest for 30 seconds and repeat this sequence 6 times. Always end with an additional exercise for the lungs. While this entire sequence, once mastered, should take no longer than 15 minutes, expect to spend 30 minutes a session as you learn to do it properly.

SIXTH WEEK AND BEYOND

By this time, daily *Chi Kung* will have become a habit. Repeat the Fifth Week sequence at least 4 times a week.

CHI KUNG FOR YOUR FACE

This technique is not just a relaxing and calming technique; it also works wonders to clear your sinuses and reduce wrinkles on your face and neck. The increased circulation works to prevent premature graying of hair and, by nourishing the follicles, decreases hair loss and gives hair a healthy glow.

Steps:
1. Sit or stand upright, taking care to relax your shoulders and back. Hold your head high and look straight ahead.
2. Rapidly rub hands together in opposite directions to generate warm *chi* energy.
3. Relax jaw.
4. Massage both sides of the bridge of your nose with your fingertips to

help circulation. This will clear your sinuses of mucus accumulations and open the breathing passages.

5. Cup the palms of your energized hands and gently press them to your cheeks, over your eyes, neck, forehead, and chin, holding them for a few seconds at each point to distribute warming *chi* energy to your face. This helps to calm muscles and nerves and stimulates energy to help eliminate wrinkles.

6. Put hands together again and rapidly rub them together in opposite directions to generate warm *chi* energy.

7. Place palms on forehead with your fingers resting on your head. Let your fingers rest on your hairline for a few seconds and then guide hands and fingers up and all the way to the back of the head a few times to guide the flow of energy through the scalp.

QUICK RELAXING CHI KUNG

I do this exercise anytime, anywhere, especially when I feel tension in my head and neck. It helps me rejuvenate when I travel on long flights. It is also very good to do before bedtime, as it can help you relax and get a good night's sleep.

Steps:
1. Sit up straight in a chair or on the side of your bed. Center your body over your hips with your knees bent and relaxed. Keep your feet flat on the floor. You should feel as if your spine is lightly suspended by a string through the top of your head.

2. Rapidly rub your palms together in opposite directions to create warm *chi* energy.

3. Place your palms over your ears with your fingertips pointing toward the back of the head. Hold for a few seconds.

4. Relax your jaw and focus on breathing deeply into the center of your body.

5. Keeping your hands over your ears, slowly tuck your chin to your chest.

Keep your elbows close to your body. Take slow, deep breaths for about a minute.

6. Slowly raise your head and elbows so that your elbows are parallel in front of your face. Keep your hands at ear level, but now move them about 3 inches from your ears.

7. Gently place your fingertips on your hairline at the nape of your neck. Lower your head slightly forward and gently tap your fingertips—like playing scales on a piano—on the lower part of your head and neck. Do this for about a minute.

8. Slowly lower your arms and raise your head. Let your shoulders relax and ease your arms to your sides.

9. Slowly and deliberately roll your shoulders up, back, and down a few times while breathing deeply and slowly.

For anyone who works at a desk or in front of a computer screen for long periods of time, take a minute or two every few hours to help release tension and keep *chi* flowing throughout the day. You'll find that your ability to concentrate is vastly improved and, as a bonus, eyestrain diminished.

You may also find that the *Chi Kung* for the Face and Quick Relaxing *Chi Kung* that I've just described are good ways to cool down after a full exercise session.

I'm sure that once you have integrated a *Chi Kung* routine into your beauty-wellness program, you will come to rely on your ability to cultivate and transform the *chi* energy of your body, mind, and spirit to empower your whole life.

11.

WEIGHTY MATTERS

BALANCE YOUR DIET AND ENERGY

AND FIND YOUR IDEAL WEIGHT

In China, weight issues are viewed in a very different light than they are here in the West. Nobody counts calories, goes on fad diets, or fasts to become thin. The Chinese believe that being overweight is simply another indication that the body is out of balance. As is being underweight. A woman's body will settle into its appropriate weight level once balance is restored and then maintained in the system.

Perhaps this cultural quest for balance explains why there is so little obesity in China. I don't remember seeing overweight people when I was growing up in Hong Kong, nor do I recall seeing any painfully thin people either. To the best of my memory—which I've verified with my sisters and parents—most people were rather average. The truth is, the only overweight Chinese people I've ever seen live in the West and, no doubt, eat a more Western diet.

As I discussed in Chapter 3, the typical Chinese diet is simple compared to the Western diet. It contains 40 to 60 percent grains and pulses, 20 to 30 percent fruits and vegetables, and only 10 to 15 percent meat, poultry, seafood, fats, and dairy products.

SWEETS FOR THE SWEET

I was shocked when I first came to the United States and saw how Americans ate. My family and I were taken out to a traditional American restaurant by friends of my parents. I saw people eating plates of food with pieces of meat large enough to feed a whole family in Asia. Before then, I had only eaten the Chinese way—a little meat stir-fried with vegetables and served with rice or some other grain.

I was also surprised at how much Americans enjoy supersweet drinks and desserts. Soft drinks and sodas tasted like colored sugar water to me. The first time I ate a piece of American cake, I thought I had bitten into a chunk of sugar. I couldn't eat it; it was too sweet for me. However, I did like the desserts I found in Europe when I went there for my modeling assignments. These pastries, cakes, pies, and tarts were not nearly as sweet as those in America.

Don't get me wrong, the Chinese also have sweet foods. Sweet soups, for example, are common (the recipe for one of my favorites—Sweet-Potato Soup—is on page 65). But the Chinese are so conscious of what is healthy to put into their bodies that almost all Chinese dishes are intended to be good for something, including the sweet soups. You'll find honey and Chinese red dates in teas, soups, and stir-fried main dishes both in Chinese cuisine and in herbal medicine.

I was in the sixth grade when my family moved to New York from Hong Kong. One day at recess, a girl asked me to hold her package of pink bubble gum so she could play ball. She offered a piece to me, too. I'd never had this treat before, so I tried it. The gum was so sweet I wanted to wash out my mouth, but I just kept chewing, trying to understand why everybody seemed to love this pink rubbery stuff. A few minutes later, my new friend came back and asked me for another piece of gum. Since she had just put some in her mouth, I asked her what happened to the bubble gum she had started chewing. She shrugged and said, "Not sweet enough." I've known since then that I would never get used to such sweetness. I've met many Americans who are addicted to sugar, who have serious problems because of their *need* to have sweet foods and drinks. This "sweet tooth" is a bad habit and is very hard to break.

During my early modeling days in New York, a friend who ate ice cream every day confided that he thought he might be addicted. He said that he felt ill if he didn't eat it. I suggested that if he really wanted to quit eating so much ice cream he should slow down and work his way out of it. He could start by eating it every other day, then every three days . . . then only on Sunday or one day a week. He thought about my suggestion and, after many attempts, was able to wean himself from his pint-a-day ice-cream habit. Now, years later, he tells me that he occasionally has a scoop of ice cream on special occasions, something that seemed impossible at first. Best of all, he has more energy and feels much better than before. I say this to let you know that anyone can break the sugar habit, and you might one day wonder how *you* ever abused your body this way.

There are many negative aspects to processed sugars, which we consume in the form of ice cream, candies, cakes, sugary soft drinks, juices, teas, and so on. Apart from the empty calories, they are known to cause mood swings and attention deficit problems. I mention this as a caution to parents who often reward their children with sweets when they do well. Children learn to associate winning and achievement with sweets, so when they grow up, they might reward themselves a little too much! Who doesn't know someone who reaches for the candy box or cake to be "sweet" to themselves?

In recent years, many people have gravitated toward low-fat and fat-free foods in an effort to stay healthy and reduce the risk of heart disease. The intent may have merit, but often the result is unexpectedly negative. You see, fat in foods—especially baked goods—contributes to the taste and texture of that food. When something is removed—in this case, the fat—something has to be added to replace it. The ingredient most often used to replace fat is sugar, especially honey and fructose, which have humectant properties that keep food moist. This moisture and texture make food feel right in the mouth and, as a consequence, taste "right."

A MATTER OF FAT

Some fat is absolutely necessary for the body to be able to digest and metabolize nutrients. Too much fat in the body interferes with the correct and natural movement of *chi* and fluids, especially through the digestive tract. This often results in heart disease, diabetes, and obesity.

The most effective way to prevent fat buildup in the body is to avoid consuming it in large quantities in the first place. Start out by removing any excess fat from meat or poultry before cooking, and certainly before eating. Chinese cooks first put meat, especially pork, beef, and even chicken, in enough boiling water to cover. Bring the water back to a boil and simmer for a few minutes. Cook a loin or roast for fifteen to twenty minutes, a chicken ten to fifteen. Then run the meat under cold water for several minutes. The fat separates from the meat and is easier to remove. This process does not destroy nutrients. Once you've done this, slice and cook the meat according to recipe directions.

According to some studies, a cup of tea can help dissolve the fat in the body. You can even marinate beef in green or black tea to remove fat, as is done in Mongolia—green tea is more effective than black tea, but either can be used. If tea is not used in cooking, make sure you drink at least one cup—the stronger, more bitter, the better—after a heavy meal to help you lose weight and reduce fat.

The Chinese drink a very potent tea called Kung Fu Cha or Kung Fu Tea, which can be found in any Chinese grocery. Like espresso in the West, it is served in tiny cups after meals. The Chinese drink it to help digestion and to help break down and eliminate fat in the body.

GET MOVING!

The most important way to balance your body's weight is to have self-discipline. Find a good exercise program that you enjoy. This can be walking with your favorite music, jogging, skating, biking, anything. Work out at the gym or stay home and do your aerobics with Jane Fonda, Richard Simmons, or Kathy Smith on video, even pick up dancing at your local dance studio. It is important that you are inspired and that what you do is fun.

Do an hour of exercise in the morning for best results, then give your body the best possible foods to nourish it at the cellular level throughout the day. Plan your meals with foods that specifically help the digestive system do its job. Pay special attention to foods that feed the stomach and spleen, and take care that you clear the stomach and intestines. Regular elimination of wastes through bowel movements will also help you get the figure you seek while beautifying the skin and hair and prolonging youth.

TAKE YOUR TIME

Sudden and drastic weight loss is not recommended. It can result in a bad complexion, including breakouts, skin irritations, or skin that is too red or too pale; lifeless hair; brittle or weak nails; weak muscles; and lack of energy and concentration. This defeats the whole purpose of losing weight to get in shape and feel good.

Believe it or not, many people who go on extremely low-calorie diets and then do not lose the weight they expect fail, in large part, because their bodies overcompensate and go into starvation mode. To conserve energy, the metabolism changes so you don't need as many calories to live on. This leaves you weak, tired, and depressed, with low immunity. Undereating also puts you in a state of emotional imbalance that can lead to irrational binge eating.

KEEP YOUR INSIDES CLEAN

As you learned in Chapter 4, detoxification and elimination play an important role in maintaining a healthy body and beauty. This is essential to weight loss. Go back to review the many ways you can help remove fat, wastes, and toxins from your body. Wastes in the gastrointestinal tract can diminish the effectiveness of the digestive process, blocking the absorption of nutrients into our bodies that actually help your body burn fat. This makes weight control difficult.

A BALANCED BODY BEGINS IN CHILDHOOD

The tendency toward obesity or extreme thinness begins in childhood. Chinese and American researchers have found that too much nourishment and an unbalanced diet during childhood can be almost as damaging to the body as malnutrition. The internal organs, especially the digestive system, develop a greater capacity for absorption and digestion than is needed to sustain health. Consequently, as the body matures, it will retain more fat and burn fewer calories. This is just another reminder that a balanced body is healthier and more fit than one out of balance. Most babies are not born overweight. It is what is put into their little systems during childhood that lays the groundwork for overweight adulthood.

A well-balanced body is exactly that. A person with a strong stomach but a weak liver is not well balanced, nor is someone who is energetic and active but has a weak heart or spleen. When one organ is excessively strong, it may cause damage to another organ. That is why all organs, all systems of the body, need to be equally nourished. According to Chinese physicians, when the stomach and spleen—the organs governing weight and digestion—are overnourished, they weaken the kidneys and bladder, inhibiting the natural elimination of water and wastes. When the kidneys and bladder are overnourished, the lungs and large intestines suffer. When the lungs and large intestines are overnourished, the liver and gallbladder are weakened. When the liver and gallbladder are overnourished, the stomach and spleen become weak.

Weight gain and edema are conditions indicating that the flow of *chi* is blocked. Fat cells have become gorged with fluids, and the organs that eliminate fluids and toxins fail to do their jobs. This means that not only the stomach and spleen but also the liver and adrenal glands are out of balance.

FOODS TO AID WEIGHT CONTROL

Besides controlling our eating habits and adding an exercise program, we can use teas, soups, and foods to curb our appetites and rid our bodies of excess fat, wastes, and water. Ironically—to the Western way of thinking—some of these same herbs and foods are also used to stimulate the appetite and bring balance to a body that is too thin. The following foods are widely used in China to aid weight control:

BITTER MELON (ALSO KNOWN AS WINTER MELON). Used since ancient times, this vegetable has been found to help alleviate high blood pressure, fat buildup, and water retention. Its juice can also be used on the face to help fade freckles and cool red noses due to excess yang energy.

BUTTON MUSHROOMS. The common button mushroom, found in any grocery store, is a cooling yin-energy food with a slightly sweet taste. It soothes the stomach, intestines, and lungs, and is known to lower blood cholesterol.

CELERY. Neutral in energy and sweet in flavor, celery is a gentle tonic for the stomach and liver. It soothes the digestive system and stimulates waste elimination.

CORN AND CORN SILK. Frequently used by Chinese herbalists to promote urination, corn and corn silk (which is often dried and brewed like tea) has neutral energy that nourishes the kidneys and digestive tract.

CHINESE LICORICE. This sweet herb with neutral energy affects the functions of the stomach and spleen. It both stimulates and suppresses the appetite, according to your body's needs.

CHINESE RED DATES. Full of warm energy, this sweet-tasting dried fruit is widely available in Chinese markets and herb shops and can be made into an effective tonic for the spleen, *chi,* and blood. Chinese red dates have detoxifying properties and nourish the spleen and stomach.

LOTUS LEAVES. A very popular herb that is used as a diuretic in cases of water retention, lotus leaves also make a very effective spleen tonic. They have neutral energy and a slightly sweet taste. Lotus leaves are often used to help reduce water retention and fat and to lower blood pressure.

LONGANS. Also used to relieve water retention, longans bring a warming energy to the body, which improves the condition of the heart and spleen. Sweet-tasting, longans—also known as logans—are known to stimulate and suppress the appetite as the body requires.

WOLFBERRIES. A dry reddish, raisinlike berry, the wolfberry nurtures and cleanses the liver and gall bladder. It is sweet tasting and can help suppress the appetite, making it valuable in weight-control programs.

WOOD EARS. These blackish brown fungi are neutral in energy and sweet in taste. They can be made into a good tonic for the stomach and large intestines, helping the body to digest foods thoroughly.

This is just a sample of the foods that aid fitness and weight control. Add them to your diet as you achieve balance within your body, and you will begin to get into shape. These, and several other foods known for their restorative properties, are included in the following recipes.

RECIPES FOR WEIGHT LOSS

Bitter Melon Soup   (yin)

This exquisite soup helps remove toxins that create imbalance in the body and cools excess yang energy. Bitter melon, which is a pumpkin-like vegetable, has been consumed for thousands of years in China. It is a very popular gourd that helps to lower blood pressure and combat fluid retention. This is an important dish for anyone who wants to lose weight.

Makes 4 to 6 main-dish servings

> 5 dried wood ears or other black mushroom, soaked in
>   warm water for 15 minutes and drained (see NOTE)
> 2 tablespoons dried baby shrimp, soaked in warm water for
>   a few minutes and drained (see NOTE)
> 1 pound bitter melon, seeded, and cut into large chunks
>   (see NOTE)
> 1 pound lean pork or smoked ham, cut into 1-inch cubes
> Salt and pepper to taste

Bring 10 cups of water and all ingredients except seasonings to a boil in a large enamel soup pot, lower the heat to medium, and simmer for 1 hour. Add salt and pepper to taste.

NOTE: Several varieties of dried black mushrooms and dried baby shrimp are available in health food stores and Asian markets. Bitter melon is available in many gourmet grocery stores and from Asian markets.

Fresh Mushroom Tofu Soup   (yin)

This quick-cooking soup is tasty and is good for all ages. Eat this soup often to soothe the stomach and intestines. It is very good not only for those who are overweight or have too much yang energy in the body but also for those with red and swollen gums, poor appetite, or urination problems. It also helps to clear heat, ease fluid retention, quench thirst, and lower cholesterol.

Makes 4 to 5 main-dish servings

   2 tablespoons soy sauce
   1 teaspoon granulated sugar
   1 tablespoon cornstarch
   1 pound lean pork, sliced into thin, bite-size strips
   ½ pound fresh button mushrooms, cut in half or smaller as desired
   ½-inch piece ginger, peeled and sliced
   ½ pound medium-firm tofu, drained and cut into ½-inch cubes
   Salt to taste

Combine soy sauce, sugar, and cornstarch in a glass bowl. Add pork, stir well, cover, and set aside.

Bring 8 cups of water to a boil in a large enamel soup pot. Add mushrooms and ginger, and return to a boil. Add tofu and marinated meat, return to a boil, then lower the heat. Cover and simmer for 15 minutes, until pork is cooked. Add salt to taste.

Gingko Tofu Soup   (yin/yang)

Gingko nuts are often used in Chinese cooking to help bring balance to the heat energy of the body, increasing digestion and thus helping weight control. This tasty soup is balanced by the cool yin energy contributed by the dried tofu skin.

Makes 4 to 5 main-dish servings

> 1 sheet dried tofu skin, or 2 to 3 sticks dried tofu (see NOTE)
> 1 pound lean pork
> 15 to 20 gingko nuts, shelled and soaked in hot water for 10 to 15 minutes to remove inner skin (see NOTE)
> 4 cloves garlic, peeled and crushed
> 1 tablespoon soy sauce
> ½ teaspoon cayenne pepper
> Salt to taste

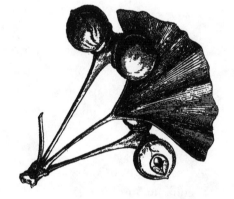

Soak dried tofu skin in hot or warm water 3 to 4 minutes until soft; drain and cut into bite-size pieces. Cut pork into 3 or 4 large pieces and put it into boiling water to cover. Boil for 5 to 10 minutes to remove fat. Rinse in cold water and drain.

Place pork, ginkgo nuts, garlic, soy sauce, cayenne, and 6 to 8 cups of water in a 4-quart enamel soup pot. Bring to a boil, then lower heat and

Gingko (*Gingko biloba*)

simmer for about an hour, until meat is tender. Add tofu skin and cook an additional 10 minutes. Add salt to taste.

NOTE: Dried tofu and gingko nuts are available at Asian markets, many health food stores, or from the mail-order Resources listed on page 253.

Chicken Liver Stir-Fry   (yang)

According to Chinese thinking, liver is a yang food that increases the burning fire of the kidneys. This increases the heat in the body, forcing it to burn up stored fat. It also stimulates the flow of chi throughout the body, making for improved digestion and elimination. Unlike traditional "diet food," this simple yet appetizing entrée appeals to the taste buds so you won't feel the least bit deprived. Chinese health experts believe that eating liver from an animal nourishes and strengthens our own liver. If liver isn't to your liking, you can use boneless, skinless chicken breasts instead.

Makes 4 main-dish servings

> 1 teaspoon salt
> 1 pound fresh chicken livers
> 2 tablespoons vegetable oil
> 3 cloves garlic, peeled and chopped
> 2-inch piece ginger, peeled and thinly sliced
> 3 to 4 scallions, cut into 1-inch pieces
> ½ cup rice wine
> Pepper to taste

Bring 3 cups of water with the salt to a boil. Add the chicken livers and cook for 1 minute. Pour off the hot water, rinse the livers in cool water, and drain.

Heat the vegetable oil till hot in a heavy wok or skillet and quickly stir-fry the garlic and ginger. Add the chicken livers and scallions and stir-fry for 3 minutes. Add rice wine, bring to a boil, and cook for 3 to 4 minutes. Add pepper to taste. Serve over rice, if desired.

Apple Seaweed Smoothie   (yin)

Another idea for anyone wanting to lose weight: Get in the habit of having an energy-packed juice drink or smoothie every day for lunch, especially during hot weather. You may feel hungry at first, but that's just your stomach telling you it's accustomed to being overfed. In a few days, you'll be used to it . . . and every hunger pang will have been worth it. Not every smoothie is sweet and sticky. Here's one that will make you feel full and satisfied. During the summer, when soup might be too hot, this juice recipe can be as good for you as it is tasty.

Makes 1 serving, approximately 16 ounces

    1 apple, peeled, cored, and cut into small pieces
    ½ medium head iceberg lettuce, cut into small pieces
    1 medium tomato, cut into small pieces
    2 tablespoons seaweed powder (see NOTE)
    Salt to taste

Place all ingredients in a blender and liquefy. Add salt to taste.

NOTE: Seaweed powder is available in Asian markets, some grocery stores, and most health food stores.

Lemon Pear Juice   (yin/yang)

This nutritious juice is cooling and energizing. A good lunch "meal" drink, it's filling, refreshing, and full of vitamins. You'll lose weight, and if you get with the program, your desired body shape will soon be yours. For variety, use different fruits.

Makes 1 serving

1 lemon, or 2 tablespoons fresh lemon juice
1 ripe pear, peeled, cored, and cut into small pieces
1 tablespoon protein powder (see NOTE)
3 or 4 ice cubes
1 teaspoon honey, or to taste

Peel and seed lemon; cut into 4 or 5 pieces. Place pear, lemon or lemon juice, protein powder, and ice cubes in a blender. Liquefy and pour into a glass. Sweeten with honey to taste.

NOTE: Protein powder is sold in vitamin shops, health food stores, and many large drugstores.

Orange Seaweed Smoothie   (yin/yang)

This powerful drink will truly energize your body, making it a welcome meal replacement for anyone wanting to lose weight. You might want to have this for lunch, when your body needs a boost.

Makes 1 serving

1 cup fresh orange juice
1 tablespoon lemon juice
2 tablespoons seaweed powder (see NOTE)
¼ teaspoon powdered ginger
2 teaspoons honey
2 or 3 ice cubes

Place orange and lemon juices in blender. Add seaweed powder, ginger, honey, and ice. Process until totally blended and smooth.

NOTE: Seaweed powder is available in some grocery stores, most health food stores, or by mail order from the Resources listed on page 253.

Grapefruit Apple Drink   *(yin/yang)*

All the ingredients in this power drink will help you lose weight. This is not a meal replacement, but it helps cut your appetite so that you'll feel fuller faster.

Makes 2 servings

> 1 apple, peeled, cored, and coarsely chopped
> 4 stalks celery, cut into 1-inch pieces
> ½ cup fresh orange juice
> ½ cup fresh grapefruit juice

Liquefy apple and celery with juices in a blender until smooth.

Water Reduction Tea   *(yang)*

Excess water is removed from the body naturally through urination and perspiration. This fragrant tea promotes both processes and warms the body to stimulate the flow of chi. *It tastes good, too! The hot energy and pungent flavor of the ginger and cinnamon cause perspiration, and the Chinese red dates and licorice provide a pleasant sweet taste and promote urination. The dried tangerine peel adds power to the brew.*

Makes 2 servings

> 2-inch piece of ginger, peeled and grated
> 10 Chinese red dates (see NOTE)
> 2 pieces Chinese licorice root (see NOTE)
> 2 cinnamon sticks
> 1-inch piece dried tangerine peel

Bring 3 cups of water to a rolling boil in a 1-quart glass or enamel saucepan. Add all ingredients. Reduce heat to low and simmer for

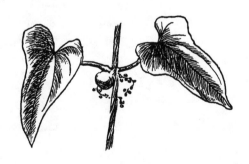

Cinnamon (*Dioscorea batatas*)

20 minutes, or until liquid has reduced to 2 cups. Strain, and drink at least twice a day.

NOTE: Chinese red dates and Chinese licorice root are available in Asian markets, in health food stores, or from the mail-order Resources listed on page 253.

Yang Tonic

As I've discussed, an important goal of the Chinese weight management program is to increase the hot (yang) energy of the kidneys. Give yang energy a boost with this remarkable tonic. Every single ingredient stimulates your kidney chi to help you get in shape. This is also a valuable tonic for people who suffer from lack of appetite.

Makes 2 servings

    3 cups water or beef broth
    4 cloves garlic, peeled and chopped
    2-inch piece ginger, peeled and grated
    5 pieces dried Chinese yam (see NOTE)
    ¼ teaspoon celery seeds

Bring water or stock to a rolling boil in a 1-quart glass or enamel saucepan. Add all ingredients to the liquid and stir. Reduce heat to low and simmer for 20 minutes or until liquid is reduced to 2 cups. Strain and drink at least twice a day.

NOTE: Dried Chinese yams look like white pieces of wood or root and are available in Chinese grocery stores, in herb shops, or from the mail-order Resources listed on page 253.

IF YOU ARE TOO THIN

The Chinese believe that extreme thinness usually results from excess hot energy and dryness. Anorexia, bulimia, or simply low body weight are believed to stem from imbalances in the bodily systems. Foods that whet the appetite and encourage balance in eating are needed to rectify this problem, which is potentially as dangerous and damaging as obesity.

RECIPES FOR WEIGHT GAIN

Chicken and Ham Soup   (yin/yang)

As appetizing as it is healthy, this hearty soup is easily digested, making it an ideal meal for anyone who suffers from lack of appetite or extreme thinness. The balanced properties of this pleasing meal help bring balance to the digestive system.
Makes 4 main-dish servings

> 1 pound boneless chicken breast, skin and fat removed, cut into
>   1-inch pieces
> ¼ pound smoked ham, cut into threads
> 1-inch piece ginger, peeled and grated
> 1 egg
> 1 teaspoon sesame oil
> Salt and pepper to taste

Bring 6 cups of water to a boil in a 4-quart enamel soup pot. Add chicken and cook over low heat for 3 to 5 minutes, until chicken turns white (almost cooked completely). Remove chicken from water with a slotted spoon, cool slightly, and mince. Reserve broth.

Add chicken, ham, and ginger to broth, and bring to a boil. Reduce temperature to low, cover, and simmer for 30 minutes. Remove from heat. Break egg into a small bowl and whisk with a fork. Slowly drizzle egg into the soup, stirring constantly to prevent clumping. Add sesame oil, then salt and pepper to taste. Return to a boil and serve.

Lamb Stew with Dang Quai (yang)

With dang quai to stimulate chi *and balance the energy in the stomach and spleen, this appetite-stimulating stew is a smart dish to serve to anyone with digestive problems. This popular dish is traditionally served to people who are extremely thin.*

Makes 4 main-dish servings

> 1 pound lamb, cleaned and cut into 1-inch cubes
> 3-inch piece ginger, cut into 3 pieces and crushed
> 4 cloves garlic, peeled and crushed
> 2 large carrots, peeled and cut into 1-inch pieces
> 1 sheet dried tofu skin, soaked for 2 minutes until soft and cut into
>   1-inch strips (see NOTE)
> 6 thin slices dang quai, approximately 3 ounces (see NOTE)
> 1 teaspoon peppercorns
> Salt and pepper to taste

Place all ingredients except salt and pepper in a 2-quart enamel soup pot with 4 cups of water. Cover and cook over medium heat for 1 hour, or until lamb is tender. Salt and pepper to taste.

NOTE: Dried tofu skin and dang quai are available at Asian markets, many health food stores, or from the mail-order Resources listed on page 253.

Chestnut Chicken Soup (yin/yang)

This soup helps strengthen the stomach and intestines, and stimulates chi *in the middle region of the body—specifically the stomach. As a result, it nurtures the entire di-*

gestive system. Besides improving the appetite, this tasty dish increases the body's ability to absorb nutrients.

Makes 4 to 5 main-dish servings

    1 pound chestnuts, shelled, skins removed, and coarsely chopped
    1 pound chicken parts, skin and fat removed
    ½ pound white button mushrooms, cut in half
    6 scallions, white part only, chopped
    1-inch piece ginger, peeled and cut into thin strips
    1 teaspoon white pepper
    1 teaspoon sugar
    Salt to taste

Place all ingredients except salt into a 4-quart enamel pot with 10 cups of water. Bring to a rolling boil; reduce heat and cover. Simmer over low heat for 3 hours, until chicken falls off bones. Add salt to taste. Discard chicken bones before serving.

12.

A LIFETIME OF WELLNESS

MENSTRUATION, PREGNANCY, AND MENOPAUSE

Just as we move through the seasons of the year, we also move through different seasons or stages in our lives. As we mature, our bodies change substantially. In early childhood, boys and girls are basically alike. They have approximately the same physical strength. Yang energy is strong, and the energy difference between the sexes is minimal. This intense yang *chi,* combined with the energy generated by the foods we eat, helps develop the body. During this very active state of childhood, we are able to eat just about as much as we want to without worrying about weight gain. The danger inherent in this, however, is that bad eating habits can develop. Unless children are taught balance and moderation in how and what they eat, they can end up with eating disorders and unhealthy eating patterns.

When we reach our teens, puberty takes over. Our body chemistry, including our metabolism, changes. For women, the feminine yin qualities surge to the fore. While boys remain in a yang energy state, girls grow stronger in a quiet, internal way. Girls' bodies develop inner strength and can endure more pain, while boys' bodies grow physically stronger.

It is during adolescence that great physical changes occur. Boys become men, and girls become women. Breasts develop and the menstrual cycle begins. This is a very important time to focus on food and nutrition.

A client of mine told me that when she was ten her mother asked her pediatrician to prescribe diet pills to help her lose her "baby fat." Now in her early fifties, she is about forty-five pounds overweight and has battled weight gain her entire life. She was born prematurely, weighing less than five pounds, but by the time she was in the fourth grade she was, in her words, "the biggest kid in my class." Until that time, she sat down for every meal with heaping plates of food and the admonition to clean her plate. This combination of food quantity and guilt laid the foundation for a serious weight problem. This woman at one time weighed almost 350 pounds.

Parents need to do everything possible to serve balanced meals to their children during childhood and adolescence, making sure that they eat as few unhealthful foods as possible. Parents must also instill good eating habits, teaching their children to eat fewer cool or cold-energy foods, or junk foods with empty calories and few nutrients. Drinking sodas or eating foods of this type will weaken the health of the stomach. Picky eaters may not get enough nutrients from the foods they *do* eat, and because their bodies are still developing, might not have the normal, healthy growth they need. By the time a child reaches puberty, he or she will not have what it takes to become a healthy adult.

The major female life cycles are menstruation, pregnancy, and menopause. Each is different, each is important, and while each can be said to control our lives, we can control these cycles as we move through them by diet, exercise, and attitude.

MENSTRUATION

A regular menstrual cycle—normal, on time, and pain free, is a sign of good health. Blood production and circulation are in order. Anything else—irregularity, pain at any time during the cycle, light or heavy flow—is indicative of imbalance. Stress, emotional upset, poor eating habits, and overactivity are some of the factors that can lead to stagnant or inadequate *chi* or irregular menstrual cycles.

Women begin menstruation in their early teens, usually between the ages of ten and fifteen. Menstruation is a mark of puberty that usually begins with the development of breasts and growth of pubic and underarm hair. It's a healthy sign of maturity and a signal that the female can become pregnant. Until the cycle is established, these early periods may be irregular in both occurrence and flow. This settling process may take only a few months or as long as a year. Once development is complete, the menstrual cycle should be normal, every twenty-one to twenty-eight days or so. Chinese doctors agree that menstruation occurs in a cycle much like the cycle of the moon; however, they do not agree with the Western way of thinking that what's normal for one woman may not be normal for another. They are alert to signs of imbalance, which they see as indicative of illness. While menstruation itself is a normal condition for women, chemical changes in the body cause many women to experience such symptoms as breast tenderness, bloating, lower back pain, even headaches and stomachaches. Any of these symptoms may indicate stagnant *chi* in the body.

WHAT'S A GIRL TO DO?

During menstruation, it's a good idea to hold back on strenuous exercise. Instead, get mild exercise and plenty of rest. Chinese tradition holds that a woman should bathe or shower more often during her period; this helps to improve circulation and relaxes muscle tension. Bathing not only makes you feel cleaner and fresher but also discourages bacterial growth. A healthy cycle and strong flow will not cause anemia, but it is best if you don't stimulate the menstrual bleeding by drinking alcohol and smoking.

I suggest that you take a look at your menstrual cycle for three or four months before your next gynecological examination so that you can be aware of what's *really* happening with your body. Describe your flow—is it spotty, heavy, thin and pale, thick, irregular, painful, or simply uncomfortable? How do you feel before, during, and after your period? Are you hot and irritable, cold and weak, phlegmy (filled with mucus), or bloated and depressed?

Once you have identified these symptoms, you will be able to use the appropriate herbal tonics to stimulate or unblock the flow of *chi* and restore balance.

You will want to eat foods that relieve discomfort and bring the body back into balance and avoid foods that increase unpleasant symptoms.

If your menstrual flow is thin, light red in color, and only lasts for two or three days, your body is exhibiting signs of a deficiency in yang or warm energy. You will probably notice that your tongue is pale, too. In this case, you will want to make sure to eat foods that stimulate *chi* and increase the warming yang energy. Eat more red beans, black-eyed peas, brown sugar, Chinese red dates, black dates, grapes, longans, pork, liver, and chicken. Avoid foods that are fried, have excessive hot energy, or are high in salt. Also limit raw foods, as they are often difficult to digest.

On the other hand, your cycle may be "normal," coming every twenty-one to twenty-eight days, but the flow may be heavy and dark and it may last for six or seven days as opposed to the more routine four or five. Chinese practitioners view these symptoms as indicative of a hot yang-energy syndrome. To relieve this, eat foods and drink tonics that help put out the fire and cool the blood— watermelon, mussels, tofu, fish, corn, bananas, tomatoes, peanuts, duck. Avoid all fried and barbecued foods, and foods that are especially spicy, such as curries and chili. Avoid smoked fish, lamb, beef and chicken, mangoes, eggs, dates, and the like, as they have too much hot energy or yang *chi* for your body to handle during this time.

PMS ALERT

One of the least understood problems women may have is premenstrual syndrome—PMS. It can last for a few days or a few weeks every month. Symptoms of this roller-coaster ride of emotions and hormones range from crankiness and moodiness, fatigue, restlessness, disorientation, and loss of focus to deep depression, fluid retention, cramps, bloating, breast tenderness, and violent mood swings. The degree of suffering depends upon which of the Five Elements are involved.

Generally, the earth and wood elements work together, affecting the organs associated with each (see page 29). When the earth element is deficient, the functions of the spleen and pancreas may be weakened. The *chi* energy to these organs is insufficient. This results in an imbalance in blood sugar and a loss of focus and concentration. When the wood *chi* is weak or stagnant, the liver and gallbladder are out of balance. This causes loss of calcium in the body, which results in muscle weakness, heart palpitations, nervousness, shakiness, and spaciness or inability to focus. The blockage of *chi* to these organs also results in fitfulness or anger.

Many people experience intense food cravings—especially for sweets and spicy foods—because of these imbalances. These cravings can be so intense that they might be better described as food addictions. Sugar cravings indicate weak *chi* in the earth organs, the stomach and spleen. Cravings for hot and spicy foods correspond with inflammation and irritation of the wood organs, the liver and gallbladder.

To alleviate the symptoms of PMS, avoid oily and fried foods, hot and spicy foods (including garlic), alcohol, caffeine, wheat, and processed sweets. Instead, eat more neutral-energy foods during this time, and eat cooling foods on a regular basis that will ease the heat energy causing your discomfort—green tea, apples, fennel seeds, caraway seeds, radishes, mint, strawberries, watermelons, mussels, fish, and tofu. Try drinking Basic Ginseng Tea (page 62) or Wild Orchid Tea (page 64) for relief. Or try any of the following recipes.

RECIPES TO EASE MENSTRUATION

Little Red Bean and Carp Soup   *(yin/yang)*

This wonderfully tasty fish and bean soup is helpful in controlling pre- and post-menstrual bloating and cramps. Little red adzuki beans promote fluid circulation and elimination, while peanuts serve as a tonic for the blood and spleen. Black-eyed peas nurture and strengthen the spleen and kidneys and also decrease fluid retention. Carp serves to strengthen the spleen, relieve edema, energize the blood, and clear the meridians for your chi. Pregnant women and new mothers will also find this dish helpful. It even promotes milk production! If this soup is too bland for your taste, add carrots, onions, turmeric, basil, or anything else that whets your appetite.

Makes 6 main-dish servings

> 1 tablespoon vegetable oil
> ½-inch piece ginger, peeled and cut into thin strips
> 1 pound carp or other white-fleshed fish fillet, cut into 2-inch pieces
> ¼ cup dried adzuki (red) beans, washed and soaked overnight
>   (see NOTE)
> ¼ cup dried black-eyed peas, washed and soaked overnight (see NOTE)
> ¼ cup raw peanuts, shelled and skins removed
> Salt to taste
> ¼ teaspoon cayenne pepper, to taste

Heat the vegetable oil in a heavy skillet. Lightly brown the ginger, remove from pan, then pan-fry fish to golden brown. Drain on paper towels.

Bring 10 cups of water to a rolling boil in a 4-quart enamel soup pot. Add beans, peas, and ginger; return to a boil. Reduce heat and simmer for 30 minutes. Add peanuts and fish. Continue cooking over low heat until beans and nuts are soft. Add salt and pepper to taste.

NOTE: For quick soaking, put beans and peas in a glass or enamel saucepan, cover with water an inch deeper than the beans, and bring to a rolling boil. Let sit for 30 minutes. Drain and cook according to recipe.

PMS-Prevention Fruit and Tofu Salad   (yin)

This is hardly a Chinese dish, but it is a recipe that follows Chinese principles. This salad is very calming to anyone who suffers the ravages of PMS. Tofu brings a bonus to the table. Made of soybeans, it includes a natural phytoestrogen that helps to stabilize the reproductive system.

Makes 4 main-dish or 6 side-dish servings

1 ripe pear
1 apple
4 large strawberries
1 ripe mango
½ pound block firm tofu
Lettuce leaves, optional

Salad Dressing
6-ounce container low-fat yogurt
2 tablespoons orange juice
1 teaspoon fennel seeds

Wash fruits. Peel pear and apple if desired. Core pear and apple and cut into bite-size cubes. Remove stems from strawberries and cut in half. Peel mango, remove seed, and cut into bite-size cubes. Place all fruits in a large glass bowl.

Press excess moisture from firm tofu. Cut into ½-inch cubes. Add to fruit bowl and toss to blend. Cover with plastic wrap and refrigerate while making salad dressing. In a small glass bowl, whisk yogurt, orange juice, and fennel seeds together. Pour over fruit and tofu mixture and toss gently to blend.

Serve on lettuce leaves if desired.

Cramp-Fighting Tea *(yin/yang)*

One of the most powerful female herbs in the Chinese herbal tradition is dang quai. A powerful tonic that strengthens chi *in the stomach and spleen, it equalizes female hormones, making it useful in treating cramps, regulating menstrual flow, and relieving other symptoms of PMS. The slightly bitter taste of the dang quai is sweetened by the addition of Chinese red dates, which improve the circulation of* chi, *and fennel seed, which has cramp-stopping and diuretic properties.*

Makes 2 servings

1-inch piece dang quai (see NOTE)
10 Chinese red dates (see NOTE)
1 teaspoon fennel seeds

Bring 3 cups of water to a rolling boil in a 1-quart glass or enamel saucepan. Add all ingredients. Reduce heat to low and simmer for 20 minutes, or until liquid has reduced to 2 cups. Strain, and drink at least twice a day to ease cramps.

NOTE: Dang quai and Chinese red dates are available in Asian markets, herb shops, or from the mail-order Resources listed on page 253.

Cardamom-Mint Tea   (yin/yang)

Cool your body's fires with this gentle, calming tea. Both cardamom seeds and mint leaves work well to encourage the flow of chi through your stomach and spleen, while removing toxins from the liver and gallbladder.

Makes 1 serving

1 tablespoon dried mint
4 to 6 cardamom seeds
Honey to taste

Bring 1½ cups of water to a boil in a glass or enamel saucepan. Add mint leaves and cardamom seeds. Return to a boil; reduce heat to low. Cover and simmer for 5 minutes. Sweeten with honey to taste. Drink warm.

Pineapple-Strawberry Smoothie (yin/yang)

Here's a cooling fruit drink that will ease the symptoms of PMS, cooling the hot energy in your system. The sweetness of the fruits helps regulate your blood sugar and, consequently, quell your cravings. The protein powder makes this tasty shake suitable for breakfast.

Makes 1 serving

    1 cup fresh pineapple cubes, canned pineapple pieces, or crushed
        pineapple
    4 to 6 medium fresh strawberries
    1 tablespoon protein powder
    3 to 4 ice cubes

Place all ingredients in the jar of your blender and process until frothy.

PREGNANCY

This part of the book is especially important to me. My pregnancy was extremely easy; however my friend Susan, who was pregnant at the same time, had a terrible time. She desperately searched for solutions to stop her morning sickness, almost constant heartburn, heavy saliva production, and loss of appetite. Except for antacid tablets, which she chewed nonstop from the time she crawled out of bed, any medication prescribed to stop the nausea made the symptoms worse. The smell of food turned her stomach; everything she ate or drank was too bitter or nauseating. She could keep two foods down—zucchini, lightly grilled without oil or salt, and salt-free soda crackers. This lasted until her seventh month. According to traditional Chinese medicine, she had a weak stomach and spleen before she became pregnant. Her pregnancy merely brought it out, just as pregnancy brings on diabetes in women who have weak pancreas and kidney function before they are pregnant. In general, these symptoms disappear after pregnancy.

Not everyone has such a bad time.

My model friend Ann was unbelievable. She gained only eighteen pounds and eight of those were her beautiful, healthy baby boy. She worked out at the gym almost daily, just as she had done before her pregnancy. With her obstetrician's supervision, she and her trainer developed a program designed to keep her fit while protecting her baby. Ann listened to her body and did everything carefully and in moderation. She was out on modeling assignments a week after her baby was born.

My friend Marsha is a runner. She was in her forties, late in her childbearing years, when she became pregnant. During her first trimester, she replaced her runs with walks and, with her doctor's approval, resumed short runs in the second trimester. She maintained her exercise program throughout her pregnancy.

Both Ann and Marsha ate sensibly before they were pregnant, so maintaining healthful eating habits during their pregnancies was easy. Both had their pre-pregnancy figures back in no time.

EATING DURING PREGNANCY

Most women don't pay much attention to their eating habits until they get ready to have a baby or, as often happens, until they're already pregnant. Many will work out at the gym, drink low-fat milk, and keep a lean diet because they don't want to fall into the "lose weight later" syndrome; they quickly bounce back to their good figure. It is important to maintain your activity—and exercise—level and establish good eating habits during your pregnancy.

If you're a healthy eater—and I do not mean "big" eater here—you're giving your baby a healthy start. As the Chinese say, all things in moderation. Health practitioners in the East and the West stress the importance of maintaining a healthy, balanced body throughout your life. They agree that this is especially true during a woman's childbearing years so that her body will be able to nurture and support a new life in the womb.

GET OFF TO A SAFE AND HEALTHY START

Check with your doctor early, ideally when you decide that you want to have a baby. If that's not possible, see your doctor or health-care practitioner as soon as you suspect that you're pregnant. A nutritious diet and appropriate fitness program will start you on your way to a safe and healthy delivery.

Pregnant women in the West are fortunate, since most will be well informed by their doctors about nutrition and exercise. There are numerous books about pregnancy, as well as plenty of support from organizations such as hospitals, insurance companies, even community centers and churches. Ask your doctor or nurse-midwife to refer you to childbirth and parenting classes. Ask friends what they did; don't just listen to their horror stories. Women considering breast-feeding their newborns might contact their local La Leche League for information and support even before their babies are born. This way, they will be able to make an informed decision about this important part of your baby's life.

During pregnancy, the baby inside you relies on your body to supply all the nutrients it needs to develop every part of its body—all the key organs, brain, muscles, tissues. Because your baby takes what it needs for growth from you, you need to have sufficient vitamins, minerals, and other nutrients for the both of you. If you don't, both you and your baby will pay the consequences.

Pregnant women used to be told that they were "eating for two." This is true . . . but only up to a point. You *do* need additional vitamins and minerals during pregnancy so that you and your baby will be healthy and strong. What you *don't* need are a lot of extra calories and fats.

During pregnancy, your appetite will change. Your senses of taste and smell will be intensified. You may experience nausea in the first three months, after meals, or any time at all. You've heard about those odd food cravings—strawberry ice cream and pickles, ketchup and jelly on everything. At times, it seems that every cell in your body is on the baby's schedule, and your hormones seem to be running amok. To ease this turmoil, try to eat small meals several times a day. Make sure that they are nutritionally balanced. Eat fewer foods with cold or cool energy.

Morning sickness is not a given. According to Chinese theory, nausea and vomiting occur when the stomach and spleen are weak and the stomach and liver are out of sync. Food is not able to pass through the digestive tract because of stagnant *chi*. If you suffer from morning sickness, this condition probably existed before the pregnancy; however, with the profound changes of pregnancy, it becomes more pronounced. You will probably feel tired and weak—always sleepy. Your tongue will be pale with a white coating and may have yellow "fur" on it. Your vomit may have a sour or bitter taste—a sure indication that your stomach and liver are out of balance. You may have a feeling of fullness or pressure in your chest and be quite thirsty, perhaps in hopes of removing that bitter taste from your mouth.

Rather than resorting to medications, I recommend these very effective drinks to settle your stomach and stop the nausea. You might want to keep un-salted soda crackers on your nightstand and eat one before getting out of bed in the morning.

RECIPES THAT EASE PREGNANCY PROBLEMS

Morning-Sickness Relief   (yin/yang)

Perfectly safe for you and your baby, this is an important recipe for pregnant women who suffer from nausea and vomiting. These conditions are caused by weakness in the stomach and spleen. Sip this gentle ginger and sugarcane-juice drink for relief. Mix a batch and keep it in the refrigerator so you can use it as needed.

Makes 8 ounces

> 1 tablespoon ginger juice (see NOTE)
> 8 ounces sugarcane juice (see NOTE)

Mix the juices together. Keep tightly sealed in a bottle in the refrigerator until needed. Sip slowly as needed to relieve nausea. You probably won't need more than half a glass.

NOTE: Ginger juice and sugarcane juice can be found in most health food stores. Simple syrup, made of granulated sugar and water, does not have the nutritional properties of sugarcane juice.

Warm Ginger Milk   (yin/yang)

Another drink that will ease nausea, Warm Ginger Milk calms the spleen and stomach. It's good for morning sickness, whatever time of day the nausea hits.

Makes 1 serving

8 ounces milk

1 teaspoon to 1 tablespoon ginger juice

In a glass or enamel saucepan, heat milk with ginger juice to taste until it begins to bubble; don't let it boil. Stir frequently to prevent sticking. Drink warm.

Dried Black Plum Tea *(yin/yang)*

The combination of dried black plums, ginger, and brown sugar neutralize the bitter nausea that results from blocks and imbalances in the stomach and liver. If you have a bitter taste in your mouth, this tea will give you almost immediate relief.

Makes 1 serving

½-inch piece ginger, or to taste, peeled, cut into 3 pieces and crushed

2 dried black plums (see NOTE)

1 tablespoon brown sugar, or to taste

Place all ingredients in a glass or enamel saucepan with 2 cups of water and bring to a boil. Reduce heat and simmer for 10 to 15 minutes, until liquid is reduced by half. Strain and add more sugar if desired. Drink warm.

NOTE: Dried black plums are available in health food stores, Asian markets, or from the mail-order Resources listed on page 253.

FOR THE SAFETY OF YOUR BABY

Everything you put in your mouth is passed directly on to your baby through the placenta. Therefore, generally speaking, all drugs and most herbs, especially medicinal herbs, should be avoided during pregnancy, even if you only *think* you might be pregnant. An example of how a good and helpful herb could end your pregnancy is *tienchi,* an herb that is most often sold in capsules and is frequently used to regulate menstrual blood flow and cramping. Do not use this herbal drug if you are trying to become pregnant or if you think you are pregnant. Tienchi will treat an embryo as just another blood clot and will flush it out of your body. Alcohol, nicotine, preservatives, food coloring, and artificial sweeteners are passed on to your baby and can cause illness and possibly birth defects. Likewise, if you get a cold or the flu when you're pregnant, your unborn baby suffers right along with you. Therefore you must take precautions so that you don't get sick. Eat well, take the vitamins and supplements your caregiver prescribes, and get plenty of rest. If you become ill, treat it yourself *nutritionally* rather than medicinally, according to Chinese practice.

Eat foods that are high in nutrients and easy to digest: soybeans, soymilk, tofu, and other soy products; lean pork; green vegetables such as spinach and bok choy; tomatoes; and fruits such as pears, apples, oranges, mandarins, tangerines, and grapes.

At least during your first trimester, avoid raw foods, other than fruit, and foods that are excessively cold in temperature, like ice cream and iced drinks and foods. Chinese research has shown that too much cold can cause miscarriage early in pregnancy. Spicy foods, such as chili and curries, should also be avoided. Later in your pregnancy you'll be able to add these foods—in moderation—to your diet if you desire.

RELIEVE WATER RETENTION

During the second trimester of pregnancy, water retention can be a problem. You may notice that your face is puffy and your fingers so swollen that you can't get your rings on and off; your feet may be so swollen that you can't get your shoes on. While pregnancy-related edema, or swelling, is not generally dangerous, it does bear watching as it has the potential to cause the baby harm. Ask your obstetrician about this.

Water retention is evidence of a yang deficiency in the spleen and kidneys. If you have weak stomach and spleen *chi,* or have eaten too much raw, cold food, spleen *chi* can be interrupted. This leads to poor water circulation in your body and you become bloated—especially in your face and limbs. The Chinese focus on strengthening the spleen and warming the kidneys to relieve edema. Eat foods with yang energy to help dispel water and swelling. Always remember to care for the baby inside you by eating foods that are warming rather than drying and cooling.

Recommended foods include rice, noodles, adzuki beans, bitter melon, lean pork and ham, liver, and chicken.

Avoid cold, raw, greasy, oily, and salty foods, as they can interrupt the spleen and kidney *chi*. Also avoid foods that are too warming—such as coffee, alcohol, curry, hot chilis, smoked fish—as they can overstimulate your unborn baby.

Bitter Melon Fish Soup   *(yin/yang)*

Bitter melon helps detoxify the system, easing the bloating caused by fluid retention during pregnancy. The use of ginger, red pepper flakes, and sesame oil bring enough hot energy to this dish to make it an especially helpful meal for a mother-to-be.

Makes 3 main-dish servings

> ½ pound fish fillets (flounder, carp, whitefish, etc.), cut into 2-inch pieces
> ½ pound bitter melon, seeds removed, and cut into 2-inch pieces (see NOTE)
> 2 stalks celery, cut into 2-inch pieces
> 1-inch piece ginger, peeled and thinly sliced
> ½ teaspoon dried red pepper flakes
> 1 tablespoon soy sauce
> ½ teaspoon sesame oil

Place all ingredients into a 2-quart enamel soup pot and add 5 cups of water. Bring to a boil; reduce heat and simmer 20 to 30 minutes, until fish is cooked.

NOTE: Bitter melon is available at Asian markets and some specialty grocery stores.

Peanut–Red Date Soup *(yang)*

Another spleen tonic, this soup increases the yang energy in the spleen and supports kidney function to relieve edema without endangering your baby.

Makes 4 main-dish servings

½ cup adzuki (red) beans
1 tablespoon vegetable oil
3 to 4 cloves garlic, peeled and chopped
½ pound raw peanuts, soaked in hot water and shaken to remove skins
12 Chinese red dates
½ pound fish filet (carp, flounder, etc.), cut into 2-inch pieces
½-inch piece ginger, peeled and sliced into 3 pieces

Wash adzuki beans and, in a 1-quart glass or enamel saucepan, cover beans with water and bring to a boil. Reduce heat and simmer 15 minutes. Drain water from beans and discard.

Heat oil in a 2-quart enamel soup pot. Quickly stir-fry garlic; stir in peanuts. Add red dates, beans, and 6 cups of water. Bring to a boil; reduce heat and simmer for 1 hour, or until peanuts and beans are almost soft enough to eat. Add fish and ginger. Return to a boil; reduce heat to medium and continue cooking for 30 to 45 minutes, until fish is cooked through and peanuts and beans are soft.

CONSTIPATION

Another problem in pregnancy is constipation. From the start of your pregnancy, make sure that you maintain regular bowel function by eating a balanced diet that includes plenty of vegetables. This is important because during your later months, usually from six months on, as the baby is growing and sitting on the intestines, normal bowel function can be disrupted. Refer to Chapter 4, where I introduce Chinese methods for treating problems with constipation.

FOR NURSING MOTHERS

I gained thirty-five pounds during my pregnancy. Since I'm five feet, nine inches and weighed 123 pounds to start with, no one even knew I was pregnant until my fourth month. After Samantha was born, I did not "diet" because I was breast feeding. I just ate sensibly, as I usually do. However, I must admit that during the first few months of breast feeding, I was constantly hungry. My body wanted steak or Ginger Chicken Soup (see page 237) and rice or other filling foods. As soon as I fed the baby, I got hungry. My body needed food to produce more milk for the baby.

After I weaned Samantha, five and then a total of ten pounds dropped from my body, bringing me back to my normal weight. This happened within about two months without my going on a special diet. I was lucky because I am pretty sensitive to what my body wants and needs, and I also know what is good for me—plenty of vegetables. It's interesting that once my body went back to its normal weight, I lost my craving for red meat.

The Chinese pay special attention to the nutrition of nursing mothers. Pregnancy takes a lot out of a woman's body, and so does nursing. For both you and your child to be healthy, you need to have plenty of nutritious foods to bring balance to both bodies. While you are nursing, make sure that your baby doesn't get colic or stomachaches by avoiding raw foods and foods that are high in yin or cold energy. Refer to the food list on pages 46–47 to refresh your memory. Sorry, but this includes ice cream and iced drinks. Cold energy foods can pass to your baby and cause colic. They are simply too strong for an infant's immature digestive system. Eat plenty of foods that are balanced—there are many recipes for soups and main courses in this book that will both whet your appetite and keep you strong and healthy during this important time in your new motherhood.

To increase milk production, you'll need to eat foods that stimulate lactation—black sesame seeds, carp and other white-fleshed fish, chicken, eggs, lettuce leaves and seeds, papayas, peanuts, and shrimp. Avoid malt (as in beer, maltodextrin, malted milk), black beans, and coffee.

RECIPES FOR NURSING MOTHERS

Ginger Chicken Soup   *(yang)*

The top choice of tonic soups given to new mothers, Ginger Chicken Soup restores balance to the body while nurturing it internally. It supplies the warming energy your body needs after pregnancy and childbirth . . . and is great for anyone with cold hands and feet.

Makes 1 main-dish or 2 appetizer servings

> 1 tablespoon vegetable oil
> One 3-inch piece of ginger, scrubbed and pounded
> 1 chicken breast or 2 thighs, skinned and cut into cubes
> ½ cup rice wine
> Salt to taste

Heat oil and stir-fry ginger and chicken. Add wine and ½ cup of water. Bring to a boil and serve. Season with salt if desired.

Sesame-Salted Eggs   *(yin/yang)*

For breakfast, lunch, or a snack, nursing mothers will want to try this simple-to-make dish. Black sesame seeds have special properties that promote lactation. Eggs are packed with protein and other nutrients that support bone development in your baby. Eat an egg a couple of times a day to promote lactation.

Makes 2 servings

> 3 tablespoons black sesame seeds, washed
> 2 tablespoons salt
> 2 hard-cooked eggs

Heat a heavy frying pan over high heat. Reduce heat to low and stir-fry the sesame seeds without oil until the seeds dry and you can smell their aroma—5 to 7 minutes. Stir in salt and mix well.

Remove shells from eggs. Dip eggs into sesame salt to eat. Anyone who is producing too much milk should not eat this often, since black sesame seeds really *do* promote lactation.

Ginger Chicken   *(yang)*

This is one of the first dishes I enjoyed after my daughter was born. I was a nursing mother and needed foods that would stimulate my appetite and aid digestion. Like Ginger Chicken Soup, it not only helps with digestion, it also warms internal energy.

Makes 4 main-dish servings

> 3 tablespoons vegetable oil
> ½-inch piece ginger, peeled and cut into thin strips
> 2 garlic cloves, or more to taste, peeled and crushed
> 1 medium onion, chopped into ¼-inch pieces
> 1 pound skinless, boneless chicken breast, cut into ½-inch pieces
> 2 tablespoons soy sauce
> 1 tablespoon sesame oil
> 1 teaspoon granulated sugar
> Salt and pepper to taste
> 1 tablespoon roasted black sesame seeds

Heat the vegetable oil in a wok or a large skillet over medium-high heat. Add the ginger and garlic, and cook, stirring constantly, for 1 to 2 minutes, until the garlic is golden brown. Stir in the onion and chicken. Add the soy sauce, sesame oil, and sugar. Cook, stirring constantly, for about 5 minutes, or until the chicken is cooked through. Season with salt and pepper to taste. Remove from heat and sprinkle with roasted black sesame seeds. Toss to blend.

Serve over rice, if desired.

MENOPAUSE

Menopause is not a death sentence. It does signify a change in life . . . often for the better. Women who have feared pregnancy are freed; women who have suffered chronic PMS no longer face this monthly malady. Menopause occurs in women in their mid- to late forties or early fifties. Chemical and hormonal changes cause ovulation and menstruation to stop. This does not happen in a moment, like turning off a light. It takes time, sometimes two or three years or longer.

The Chinese believe that if you are in good health and a good state of mind you will have few problems going through this new phase of life. Menopause begins with menstrual irregularities, both in the length of your cycle and flow. About 80 percent of all women experience some symptoms—night sweats, insomnia, tiredness, excitability and edginess, dizziness, loss of focus, blurry vision, bloating, forgetfulness, increased perspiration, or hot and cold flashes. There are also emotional issues surrounding menopause, as many women mourn the loss of their fertility.

The Chinese treat the symptoms of menopause in the same ways they would other imbalances in the body, especially imbalances in the kidneys. Hot flashes are evidence of excess yang energy, which requires cooling, or yin, foods to bring relief. Vaginal dryness is symptomatic of excess yin. This condition is relieved by foods and topical products that cool the hot energy that has dried up the body's natural moisture. Some women experience both yin and yang deficiencies, which can be especially uncomfortable and stressful. Either deficiency can affect the functioning of the heart, spleen, and liver, making restoration of balance to the kidneys very important to the health and well-being of the woman.

Yin deficiencies in the kidneys can occur as dizziness, headaches, blurred vision, lightheadedness, ringing in the ears, hot flashes, excessive perspiration and night sweats, or even high blood pressure. There is often soreness in the lower body, restless, dream-filled sleep, a dry mouth, and red tongue.

Indicators of a kidney yang deficiency likewise include headaches and blurred vision, as well as lower back pain, cold limbs, intense tiredness and weakness, and restless sleep interrupted by frequent urination. There is often a loss of taste and a pale tongue. Early in menopause, irregular menstruation is common, even expected; however, when there is a shortage of yang energy in the kidneys, flow varies from heavy to sparse, with periods stopping for several months at a time.

Most of these symptoms can be relieved with a diet rich in foods that nourish the kidneys.

FOODS THAT EASE SYMPTOMS OF MENOPAUSE

Fruits and nuts: apples, apricots, bananas, cashews, coconut, figs, grapefruits, oranges (especially mandarin oranges), papayas, peanuts, persimmons, prunes and plums, walnuts, watermelons.

Vegetables: adzuki beans, broccoli, cabbage, castor beans, celery, Chinese cabbage, corn, cucumbers, eggplants, green beans, kidney beans, lentils, lettuce, parsnips, potatoes, shiitake mushrooms, snow peas, spinach, sweet potatoes, tomatoes, turnips, watercress, zucchini and other squashes.

Proteins: eggs, fish, lamb, milk, pork, tempeh, tofu, yogurt.

Grains and seeds: barley, black sesame seeds, brown rice, oats, peanuts, sunflower seeds, walnuts, wild rice.

Miscellaneous: basil, ginseng, honey, sesame oil, soy sauce.

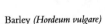

Barley *(Hordeum vulgare)*

FOODS TO AVOID

Alcohol and other red meat, Chinese parsley (coriander), coffee and other forms of caffeine, crabapples, cured meats, dairy products (except yogurt), fried and fatty foods, spicy foods, hawthorn fruits, processed or salty foods.

NATURAL ESTROGEN REPLACEMENTS

Many of the changes associated with the *cessation* of menstruation are attributed to the fact that the body no longer produces estrogen. Lower estrogen levels can cause hot flashes, vaginal dryness, dry skin, joint stiffness, arthritis, and loss of bone density, as well as hardening of the arteries. To make up for this loss, synthetic estrogen is often prescribed by Western physicians. However, the use of synthetic estrogen has its downside, specifically the increased risk of breast or uterine cancer. Even the small dose of progesterone often prescribed by Western doctors to bring balance to an estrogen replacement program has been found to result in blood clotting, gallbladder disease, asthma, and seizures.

Traditional Chinese practitioners have recorded much success in treating menopause with a variety of foods and herbs that free the circulation of body fluids while balancing *chi,* blood flow, body fluids, and hormones.

The best known of these natural estrogen-replacing foods are Mexican yams and soy foods, including tofu, tempeh, and sprouts. Others that fit easily into a balanced diet are alfalfa sprouts (great for salads), apples, barley, beets, black beans, black-eyed peas, cabbage, carrots, cashews, cherries, chickpeas, clover sprouts (another tasty salad ingredient), corn and corn oil, cucumbers, fennel, garlic, green mung beans, hops, legumes, licorice, oats, olives and olive oil, papayas, plums, potatoes, pumpkins, red beans, rhubarb, rice, sage, sesame seeds, squashes, sunflower seeds, and whole wheat. Flaxseeds and flaxseed oil—sprinkled over salad greens and blanched veggies—assist the absorption of nutrients, moisten the lower intestines, and facilitate natural estrogen replacement.

Estrogenic herbs that are part of the Chinese approach to combatting menopausal symptoms include both fresh and dry dandelion flowers, dang quai, ginkgo leaves, ginseng root, Chinese licorice root, raspberry leaves and raspberries, St. John's Wort, Chinese yam, and royal jelly.

NEWS ABOUT HOT FLASHES

For centuries, Chinese women have known about *fengwang,* or royal jelly, one of the best ways to combat the surging hot flashes commonly associated with menopause. This supernutritious food is eaten only by the queen bee, who lives twenty times longer than the worker bees in her hive. The poor worker bee lives four or five months, while the average queen lives five or six years. Her longevity is attributed to her diet, which consists solely of royal jelly. Royal jelly contains a full range of amino acids, vitamins, minerals, enzymes, and other nutrients that stimulate the queen's incredibly productive fertility. Taken internally or applied topically, the powerful nutrients in royal jelly improve elasticity, smoothing and softening the skin, so that it looks younger and fresher.

Pure royal jelly may be difficult to find unless you have access to a beekeeper. However, premixed concoctions made of ginseng and royal jelly liquid, or ginseng, royal jelly, and schizi berries, can be found in Asian markets and health food stores coast to coast. Royal jelly and royal jelly compounds are usually packaged in small brown glass vials. Take it like a vitamin or food supplement. You must use your own judgment as to how much you need and how often you need it. It is bitter, but you will immediately feel enlivened and regenerated, and your hot flashes will cool down.

FOOD FOR HEALTHY BONES

The loss of bone density associated with menopause can be slowed by a diet that supplies the body with a minimum of 1000 milligrams of calcium. This can come from calcium-enriched milk, calcium-enriched soymilk, bone meal, or calcium supplements—calcium citrate and calcium carbonate are especially easy to absorb, as is a calcium-magnesium combination. Supplements are best taken on an empty stomach and should not be taken with cereals, grains, and legumes, since these foods can reduce mineral absorption. If you have questions about how much calcium supplementation you need, consult your doctor.

While relatively high in absorbable calcium, cheese and some other milk products, including butter and margarine, are unnecessarily high in fat and, in many cases, salt. Therefore, they should be consumed in limited quantities.

Foods that are high in calcium and other minerals include salmon, tuna, sardines, oysters, apricots, figs, broccoli, and spinach and other green leafy vegetables.

EATING FOR HEALTH, YOUTH, AND BEAUTY

Vitamins and minerals are a Western concept; however, for our purposes I will use them to describe foods that keep us looking young and feeling beautiful at any age—especially before, during, and after menopause.

Animal liver and kidneys; crustaceans such as shrimp, crawfish, and prawns; oysters and other shellfish; and nuts and legumes are all necessary for healthy hair, skin, and nails. High in copper, these foods promote the production of collagen, a tough, fibrous, elastic tissue found in bone, tendons, skin, and cartilage. Collagen keeps the skin and mucus membranes moist, thick, and strong and the skeletal system more flexible. These foods are also known to ease random joint stiffness and arthritis pain.

Alfalfa, bananas, berries, broccoli, Brussels sprouts, cantaloupes, cayenne pepper (capsicum), citrus fruits, green and red peppers, green leafy vegetables, guavas, potatoes, rose hips, spinach, sprouted grains, sweet potatoes, tomatoes, and watermelons—all foods high in vitamin C—also maintain healthy collagen. When ligaments and bones are more flexible, they are less likely to be injured. Vitamin C has other age-defying properties. It is a powerful antioxidant and free-radical quencher that fights inflammation and slows down the aging process. Circulation is vastly improved by the vascular-dilating properties found in foods and supplements high in vitamin C.

Sweet potatoes and yams and other foods high in vitamin A and beta carotene help to bring balance to the liver and nourish the skin, keeping it supple and strong. Papayas, apricots, carrots, melons, tomatoes, and other red, yellow, and orange vegetables and fruits all bring moisture and balance to the skin. Vitamin E works with vitamin A to strengthen the skin and mucus membranes, reducing vaginal dryness and causing age spots to fade.

Add foods rich in vitamin D to your diet—fish liver oils, fatty fish, chicken and beef liver, egg yolks, and dairy products—to further bring balance to the liver and kidney *chi*. Deficiency of this vital nutrient promotes thinning hair, brittle nails, and rapidly aging skin. Too much of this vitamin creates an unfavorable climate that can produce kidney stones.

For longer-lasting health, vitality, and youthfulness, limit fats, salt, refined sugars, and chemical additives. Notice that I didn't say *eliminate* fats. Our bodies need essential fatty acids, which are found in polyunsaturated fats, to strengthen cell membranes and to digest and metabolize foods. Because the body is unable to manufacture these substances, and our cells cannot function normally without them, we must supplement our diet with them. Rich sources of polyunsaturated fats are safflower seeds and oils, grapeseed oil, flaxseed oil, sunflower seeds and oil, sesame seeds and oil, canola oil, olives and olive oil, and avocados and avocado oil. Other valuable sources are mackerel, herring, flounder, trout, and bass (not fried or smoked) as well as cod liver oil, shrimp, oysters, sea vegetables and seaweeds, pumpkin seeds and oil, and black currants.

In the conventional Western tradition, vitamin B complex supplements are taken for healthy skin, eyes, and hair. Foods that provide these vitamins are also known to Chinese practitioners as foods that bring balance to the flow of *chi* throughout the systems of the body, aiding in easing anxiety, sleep disruption, and lowered libido. Important sources are whole grains, organ meats, eggs, brewer's yeast, cauliflower, Brussels sprouts, and soy products, including tofu and tempeh.

Here are a few tasty recipes to keep you young, vital, and beautiful.

Honey Egg Milk   (yin)

Sip this tasty drink to relieve such symptoms of menopause as weakness, dizziness, forgetfulness, shortness of breath, sleeplessness, hot flashes, and nightsweats. You'll find it very calming to your system. Drink nightly as desired.

Makes 1 serving

> 8 ounces whole or reduced-fat milk
> 1 egg
> Honey to taste

Bring milk to the boiling point in a glass or enamel saucepan. Break egg into a saucer and whisk lightly to break the yolk. Add egg to milk and whisk over medium heat for 1 minute. Pour into a large mug and sweeten with honey as desired.

Chinese Yam and Chicken Congee *(yin/yang)*

Everyone else at your dinner table will think you've made a delicious rice soup. Only you will know you've cooked up a health-giving stew that will cool your hot flashes, ease lower back pain, and soothe irritability.

Makes 3 to 4 main–dish servings

> 2 chicken thighs, skin removed
> 5 to 7 pieces dried Chinese yam (see NOTE)
> ¼ cup rice
> ½ pound skinless, boneless chicken breast, cut into thin strips
> 2-inch piece ginger, peeled and cut into threads
> 2 to 3 cloves garlic, peeled and chopped
> 1 tablespoon soy sauce
> 1 teaspoon sesame oil
> 4 stalks celery, cut into 1-inch pieces

Bring 5 cups of water, chicken thighs, and Chinese yam to a boil in an enamel saucepan. Lower heat to medium and simmer for 30 minutes. Remove chicken thighs. Remove the meat from the bones and cut into bite-size pieces. Set aside.

Add the rice to the broth and return to a boil. Reduce heat and continue to cook over medium–low heat for about 30 minutes. Do not cover.

Place chicken breast, ginger, and garlic in a bowl; add soy sauce and sesame oil, and toss to coat. Let marinate for about 30 minutes while rice cooks.

Add the chicken slices, marinade, and celery to the rice soup; bring to a boil. Stir to prevent sticking. Reduce heat; cover pot, and continue cooking for 10 minutes. Add thigh meat and continue cooking 5 more minutes or until breast meat and rice are completely cooked.

NOTE: Dried Chinese yam is available from Asian markets and the mail-order Resources listed on page 253.

Walnut Chicken Ding   (yin/yang)

What woman wouldn't want to serve a main dish that increases sex drive? This traditional Chinese main dish does exactly that. By nurturing kidney yang energy, Walnut Chicken Ding combats weakness and tiredness and improves the sexual appetite.

Makes 2 to 3 main-dish servings

  3 tablespoons vegetable oil
  ¼ cup walnut halves
  2 to 3 cloves garlic, peeled and chopped
  2-inch piece ginger, peeled and thinly sliced
  ½ pound boneless, skinless chicken breast, cut into ½-inch pieces
  2 to 3 stalks celery, cut into ½-inch pieces
  Salt to taste

  Sauce
  1 tablespoon soy sauce
  1 teaspoon sugar
  3 tablespoons cornstarch

Heat oil in a wok or heavy skillet. Stir-fry walnuts, garlic, and ginger. Add chicken and celery, and stir-fry about 5 minutes.

  Add 1 cup of water to sauce ingredients in a 2-cup measuring cup and stir until cornstarch dissolves. Pour over chicken mixture and continue cooking for 2 to 3 minutes, until sauce begins to thicken. Add salt to taste.

  Serve over rice, if desired.

Red Date Tea   *(yin/yang)*

Chinese women drink this nutritious and tasty tea in the morning and at bedtime to calm the anxiety and jumpiness often associated with menopause. You may not feel hysterical or overly anxious, but you may certainly feel on edge during this time of great change. This simple drink will put you at ease.

Makes 2 servings

> 1 small yam, peeled and cut into ¼-inch pieces
> 6 to 8 Chinese red dates (see NOTE)
> 4 pieces Chinese licorice root (see NOTE)
> 2 tablespoons wheat germ

Place all ingredients in a glass or enamel saucepan, add 4 cups of water, and simmer for 30 minutes over medium heat, or until liquid is reduced by half. Stir occasionally. Strain liquid and drink warm or cool.

NOTE: Chinese red dates and Chinese licorice root are available at Asian markets, health food stores, or from the mail-order Resources listed on page 253.

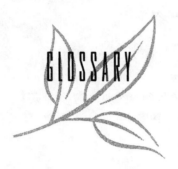

GLOSSARY

Adzuki beans or small red beans A neutral energy food, these slightly sweet beans are easily digested, making them an important part of the diet for anyone who is ill. They are also good for children and the elderly. Menstruating women will find adzuki beans, used in a soup or stew, useful in regulating flow.

Anise/star anise This warm, pungent, and sweet spice promotes the circulation of yang energy through the skin and muscles. Affecting the spleen, kidneys, and liver, it can be boiled—seven star anises and seven fresh heads of scallion in three cups water, reduced to one cup—and sipped like tea to treat constipation and detoxify the system.

Astragalus Chinese name, *Huang Chi*. An effective energy and heart tonic with a slightly warm or yang energy, this herb is known to regulate blood pressure and blood sugar, improve circulation in the flesh and skin, boost the immune system, and promote healing of wounds. Organs most affected by astragalus are the spleen, lungs, and kidneys.

Barley A versatile grain that can be used in soups and stews as well as ground to be used in exfoliating skin treatments, barley has a cooling energy that regulates digestion, promotes urination, and aids elimination.

Bitter melon Also known as bitter gourd, this soft green melon has been used since ancient times to help high blood pressure, fat detoxification, and water retention caused by various conditions, including kidney disease, heart disease, and cirrhosis. The fresh juice of this winter melon can also be applied to the face to help remove freckles and cool red noses due to excess hot energy or drunk to relieve sunstroke and thirst. The peel is commonly used in Chinese medicines with great effects.

Black sesame seeds A powerful tonic for the liver and kidneys, black sesame seeds are used to relieve dry skin, stimulate milk secretion in nursing mothers, and reverse premature graying.

Button mushrooms The common button mushroom, found in any grocery store, is a cooling energy food with a slightly sweet taste that affects the stomach, intestines, and lungs. It is known to lower blood fat. Button mushrooms are also used for their antibiotic properties.

Celery Neutral in energy and sweet in flavor, celery is a gentle cooling tonic food for the stomach and liver. It affects the digestive system and stimulates waste elimination.

Chi Life energy or life force. The breath of life.

Chicory An appetite stimulant and digestive aid, the entire chicory plant is known to stimulate the central nervous system. Organs affected by chicory are the liver and gall bladder.

Chinese licorice This sweet herb with neutral energy affects the functions of the stomach and spleen. It both stimulates and suppresses the appetite, as your body needs. An important digestive aid, licorice also dispels fever, and eases cough and sore throats. The root is known to fight bacteria, is good for skin rashes, and cleanses and heals skin sores. A potent inhibitor of acne-type skin problems, this popular Chinese herb is used as a balance to counteract any toxins or poisons in most herbal prescriptions. It benefits all organs.

Chinese red dates Full of warm energy, this sweet-tasting dried fruit is widely available in Chinese markets and herb shops. It is an effective tonic for the spleen, *chi*, and blood. It has detoxifying properties and affects the spleen and stomach.

Cinnamon The bark of the cinnamon tree is dried and used as a seasoning in many Chinese dishes. Its hot energy and pungent and sweet properties affect the kidneys, spleen, and bladder. Dissolved in rice wine, it is given to mothers after childbirth to relieve pain. Cinnamon is also used as a digestive aid. Cinnamon twigs are used to warm the body by promoting blood circulation and causing perspiration, relieving arthritis pain that is worsened when exposed to cold.

Cloves Chew one or two cloves and this warm, pungent spice gets rid of bad breath. Cloves warm the internal organs, especially the stomach, spleen, and kidneys.

Coconut and coconut milk Coconut meat has neutral energy, while the milk is warm. Both are considered important in preventing premature aging.

Corn and corn silk Frequently used by Chinese herbalists to promote urination, corn and corn silk (which is often dried and brewed like tea) has neutral energy that affects the kidneys and digestive tract.

Cucumbers An important food used to relieve acne, cucumbers have a cooling energy that relieves hot skin conditions. Applied externally, it is also used to relieve burns.

Dang quai A nutritious herb that is used to speed recovery from illness, dang quai is probably the best known "female" herb, used to ease menstrual cramps and stop diarrhea. Used to strengthen the *chi* energy in the stomach and spleen, warming these organs when they suffer from excess cold energy. Dang quai also is used as a blood tonic and is known to speed the healing process of bruises.

Fennel Fennel seeds are warm and pungent, promoting energy circulation through the kidneys, bladder, and stomach. Fennel root, which is also warm, tastes pungent and sweet. Both are used to bring warmth to the kidneys and promote circulation of energy to relieve pain.

Garlic One of the most versatile herbs used by the Chinese, garlic is a warm and pungent bulb that is known for its antibiotic properties. It affects the spleen, stomach, and lungs and is considered an aid to digestion.

Ginger An important detoxifying agent, gingerroot has warm energy that relieves nausea, disperses cold, induces perspiration, and affects the stomach, lungs, and spleen. Mixed with orange juice, grated ginger eases motion sickness. Boiled in water and steeped until the color of weak tea and sweetened with honey, ginger will warm the systems of the body and combat the symptoms of cold.

Gingko biloba Gingko nuts help balance moisture in the lungs, calm coughs, reduce phlegm (mucus) and vaginal discharge. Gingko is beneficial to heat energy throughout the body, helping to energize the blood and reducing fat. It is a mild diuretic and natural antidote for alcohol poisoning. Use gingko moderately. While it is one of the most popular nutritional herbs and is also used in everyday cooking, gingko nut contains very mild toxin, especially the middle part. Even though I've never heard of anyone's being poisoned by it, it's always a good idea to keep balance and never overeat it.

Ginseng Ginseng is considered the premiere Chinese tonic herb. *The Yellow Emperor's Classic of Internal Medicine* says, "Ginseng is a tonic to the five viscera, quieting the animal spirits, stabilizing the soul, preventing fear, expelling the vicious energies, brightening the eyes and improving vision, opening up the heart, benefiting the understanding, and, if taken for some time, will invigorate the body and prolong life." Ginseng is an energy tonic, which replaces lost *chi* to the meridians and organs. It is said to benefit the mind, soul, and spirit as well as the body. This may account for its 2000-year popularity. Most commonly available and most effective is Korean ginseng.

Honey An amazing humectant with antibiotic properties, honey brings neutral energy to the body. Affecting the lungs, spleen, and large intestine, honey eases an upset stomach, relieves constipation, and treats hypertension. Externally applied, honey relieves pain of burns and heals blemishes.

Ho Shou Wu Also known as Chinese Cornbind (Multiflower Knotweed Root), Ho Shou Wu has a slightly warm or yin/yang balance. This potato-like root nourishes blood and semen, helps constipation due to dry intestines, swelling of lymph glands, abscesses and ulcers, insomnia; and it is famous for its cure for premature greying of hair.

Longans Also used to relieve water retention, longans bring a warming energy to the body which improves conditions of the heart and spleen. Sweet tasting, longans are known to stimulate and suppress the appetite as the body needs. This herb is the meat of a small round fruit that is somewhat like lychees. The longan shell is smooth and tan color, unlike lychee shells, which are red and bumpy. Some books erroneously use the word longan to describe the wolfberry.

Lotus leaves A very popular herb that is used as a diuretic in cases of water retention, it is also a very effective spleen tonic. Lotus leaves have neutral energy and a slightly sweet taste. Lotus leaves are often used to help clear edema and fat and help lower blood pressure.

Peanuts A neutral energy food, peanuts stimulate the appetite and lubricate the lungs. Boiled with rice, peanuts make a congee that is given to nursing mothers to promote milk secretion.

Radishes This cool, pungent, and sweet root affects the stomach and lungs. Radishes are used to treat a variety of ills, from indigestion to colds and headaches. Fresh radish juice is a reliable hangover cure, and, mixed with ginger juice, cures laryngitis.

Rice Whether you're using brown rice, white rice, or glutinous sweet rice, this neutral energy grain acts as an energy tonic that affects the spleen, stomach, and lungs. A tablespoon of rice, mixed with fresh ginger juice, is guaranteed to relieve morning sickness.

Royal jelly *(fengwang)* Royal jelly is the super-nutritious food that the queen bee eats. Queen bees live twenty times longer than the worker bees. The average worker lives four to five months; the average queen bee lives from five to six years. This longevity is attributed to her diet, which consists solely of royal jelly. It contains a full range of amino acids, vitamins, minerals, and enzymes. This jelly stimulates the queen's incredibly productive fertility. Pure royal jelly is harder to find; make sure it is fresh and keep it in the fridge. Use within six months. When looking for premixed Chinese vial concoctions, look for the word *fengwang*. That means royal jelly.

Soy beans, soy bean curd The energy of soy beans and soy products such as tofu and tempeh depends upon how they are prepared. Powerful detoxifying foods, soy is used as an energy tonic, affecting the spleen, stomach, and large intestines.

Sweet potato A neutral-energy food that acts as a yin energy kidney tonic, sweet potatoes can be used in soups that calm digestion, moisturize the intestines, and, used in a sweet soup, help to ease discomfort of pregnancy.

Tofu See Soy beans.

Watermelon A food with cold energy, this sweet-tasting fruit promotes urination and lubricates the intestines. Affecting the heart, stomach, and bladder, fresh watermelon can be eaten to cure a hangover and stimulate bladder function. Watermelon peel can be dried and then boiled in water as a tea to ease hypertension, diabetes, and kidney disease.

Wolfberry A dry, reddish, raisin-like berry, the wolfberry nurtures and cleanses the liver and gall bladder. It is sweet tasting and can help suppress appetite, making it valuable in weight control programs.

Wood ear fungi This blackish-brown fungus is neutral in energy and sweet in taste. It is a good tonic for the stomach and large intestines, helping the body digest foods properly and thoroughly.

Yams A sweet, neutral-energy food, yams are used in tonics for the spleen, lungs, and kidneys. Some varieties are found to be high in phytoestrogen, while all have been found useful in regulating blood sugar levels in diabetics.

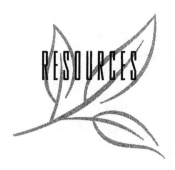

RESOURCES

MAIL-ORDER AND STORE RESOURCES

Aphrodisia Products, Inc.
(Source of oils, extracts, herbs, and spices, including some Chinese herbs)
264 Bleecker St.
New York, NY 10014
(212) 989–6440

Great China Herb Company
857 Washington St.
San Francisco, CA 94108
(415) 982–2195
Fax: (415) 982–5138

Helen Lee Spa
205 East 60th Street
New York, NY 10022
(212) 888–1233
Web site: www.helenLee.com

K&F Trading Company
44 The Bowery
New York, NY 10013
(212) 619–3298

Kam Man Food Products, Inc.
200 Canal St.
New York, NY 10013
(212) 517–0330/0331
Fax: (212) 766–0–85

Lin Sisters Herb Shop, Inc.
4 The Bowery
New York, NY 10013
(212) 962–5417
Order and Information Line:
1–888–LIN–SIST
Fax: (212) 587–8826
Contacts: Frank or Susan Lin

Superior Trading Company
837 Washington St.
San Francisco, CA 94108
(415) 982–8722
Fax: (415) 982–7786

NATIONAL CHAIN STORES AND HELP LINES

East Earth Herbs, Inc.
Stores nationally
Order and Information Line:
1–800–827–HERB

Wild Oats
Stores nationally
Help Line: 1–800–494–WILD

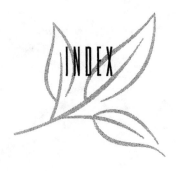

INDEX